WHEN KIDS NEED MEDS

Everything a Parent Needs to Know About Psychiatric Medication and Youngsters

HENRY A. PAUL, MD

Carnegie Hill Psychiatric Associates

35

70

105 → 75

140 → 40

175 → 75

210 → 30

245 → 65

280 → 80

Disclaimer

Information contained in this book is intended for educational purposes only. It is not intended as medical or psychiatric advice for individual conditions or treatment and does not substitute for a medical or psychiatric examination. A psychiatrist must make a determination about any treatment or prescription. The author does not assume any responsibility or risk for the use of any information contained within this book.

This book contains information about psychotropic medications and children and adolescents. Please note that recommended doses are not discussed for any particular drug. Appropriate doses are determined by each prescriber for each individual child or teenager.

ISBN-10: 146647694X
ISBN-13: 9781466476943

Library of Congress Control Number: 2011919569
CreateSpace, North Charleston, SC

This book is dedicated to my dear friend and colleague
Gordon Whitaker, LCSW.

Orion

2
4
8
10
16
24
26
30
10
40
32
36
44
48
54

64
66
76
80
84
64
56
64
68
68
0
8
4

20
28
12
0

Who is Monet?

CONTENTS

INTRODUCTION

I received the following phone calls last week:

"The school principal just called and said our son Steven, a fourth grader, was overheard talking with some friends about bringing a knife to school. He has a history of misbehavior, but recently he has gotten worse. He has been fighting a lot, not following rules, talking back, leaving the classroom without permission, and now this. I'm freaking out. When can we see you?"

"Our fourteen-year-old daughter, Jessica, has been sad since her grandma died six months ago. She's been withdrawn, sleeping a lot, and hardly eats. At first we sympathized with her and gave her space. But this morning I looked in her diary and read a note in which she talked about yearning to be dead and join her grandma in heaven. I think this is much worse than just grieving. What should we do?"

"Marty, our eleven-year-old son, has always been shy. Ever since we can remember, he was scared to do anything new. We would have to accompany him everywhere—school, camp, after school activities, and the like. He could never go on a play date without great fear. He never made close friends. But now he is beginning to act really strange. He talks to himself, he is over-involved on strange websites, he smiles about things we can't understand, and yesterday said something about being connected to other people through mindreading. I read something about psychosis on the

Internet and he seems to fit the bill. I'm terrified something really serious is wrong with him."

I get calls like these almost every day. Realizing that your child has a problem is scary. It can be devastating to learn that your child is physically sick, but discovering that your child suffers from a mental disorder adds another layer of confusion and anxiety. Mental disorders are not as well understood as physical disorders, and it is only recently that they have begun to be talked about openly. Add the fact that new diagnoses come up seemingly weekly, along with all the misinformation in the media about the medications used to treat mental disorders, and you have some very confused and worried parents. If you fall into that category, this book is for you. My goal is to address your questions, fears, and worries about giving your child or teenager medication for a diagnosed mental disorder.

Do children really suffer from mental disorders? Isn't that only the domain of adults? Unfortunately, no. It might be helpful to consider the numbers. There are approximately 75 million children and teenagers in the country. About one in five young people less than eighteen years old are thought to suffer from a bona fide mental disorder. That is at least 15 million of our youth. In that number, approximately half suffer from a serious mental health disturbance and about half of those from what is called an extreme disturbance. Thus, it is no surprise that there has been a tremendous increase in the use of psychotropic drugs—medications which seek to affect behavior, thinking, or emotions—in children and teenagers over the last several decades. Newspaper headlines describe the use of these drugs as an epidemic. Political candidates have promised to investigate the trend. Although it is difficult to quantify, the increase seems to be at least four or five fold. It is estimated that several million young people now take these drugs, and while some feel that this is too many, people in the mental health field feel that this is probably only a small percentage of those who need it. Furthermore, the numbers will only increase as diagnostic criteria are refined and medications become more available for children—two trends which have increased over the past decade.

As a prescribing child and adolescent psychiatrist, I have witnessed and participated in this virtual explosion of prescribing to children and teens. Although I am convinced of the enormous help that these medications provide if prescribed properly and in conjunction with other forms of therapy, I am also sensitive to the fears, reluctance, and questions that parents have. I am fully aware of the debates that accompany such rapid growth in the field. Questions and fears are based not only on parents' inherent and natural concerns about the welfare of their children, but also on the information—and misinformation, mainly through the media—that inundates us.

For some parents, the idea of children taking any medication can be scary. Psychotropic medications, however, seem to frighten nearly every parent. Everyday I hear anxious questions and statements from concerned parents when told that medication might help their child. Parents don't know what to do. Many have been frightened because of what they have read in newspapers and magazines or seen and heard on television and radio. Some are just opposed, while still others simply seek more knowledge before starting down the road of medication use by their child.

Recently, I jotted down the questions and comments of parents I saw in my practice. Here is a sample of what I heard:

"These drugs are harmful—we don't even know how they work."
"There is nothing really wrong with my child, it's just a bit of extreme behavior, certainly not a disorder."

"My neighbor's daughter died from that medication."
"I heard these medications are addictive."
"Antidepressants cause suicide."
"I just want to use natural remedies."
"Won't these chemicals affect my child's brain development?"
"I don't want my son to be a zombie all day."
"I'm afraid the side effects will be worse than the disorder."
"Mental disorder runs in the family. It's impossible to fix."
"Kids are kids; it's ridiculous to give their behavior a clinical name."
"Some guy on Oprah said Ritalin is just like cocaine."
"That kid on the news who killed his family was on Zoloft. They say it made him violent."
"Don't schools just want children medicated to make them easier to handle?"

From years of practice and education I have become familiar with the arguments about the use, and possible misuse, of psychotropic medication for young people. While good healthy debate helps us all, this subject has also attracted many who distort, exaggerate, and even make up stories. My participation on radio and television shows, in particular, sensitized me to the dangers of relying on sound-bite newscasts or talk show drama when it comes to terribly important topics. I have learned that many of the "experts" have had little or no experience in the trenches working with children. But because they're on television, they are assumed to be knowledgeable and so become a source of misinformation for many viewers.

One time stands out in particular: I was on a national talk show, viewed by millions of parents, talking about the medications used for attention deficit hyperactivity disorder (ADHD) with another doctor who had written a popular book against the use of any medication for this disorder. During a commercial break, I asked the author how he had become so convinced that medications are dangerous, as I had never seen many of the problems he was describing. He told me that he was not a child psychiatrist, but a family medicine practitioner for adults and had never even treated a child or teenager with ADHD. He said he had written his book based on a literature search he had done on his computer. His book was doing well and the audience warmed to his comments, as he tapped into the great anxieties that most people have about giving their children medication. I worried that parents listening to him might withdraw life-saving, school-saving, family-saving, abuse-saving medication treatments because of his biased arguments—arguments not based on fact or experience.

I have also seen well-meaning but poorly informed newscasters and talk show hosts say things that are simply not true. Studies are quoted that do not exist. Personal experiences are presented after "careful screening" of guests who will present predictable and often prejudiced, distorted, and even false personal reports that play well on television but perpetuate unwarranted fears in millions of viewers. Horror stories about a dramatic "side effect" make the front pages even if, in fact, the side effect did not happen. In the event that it did happen, no one bothers to mention that the side effect is so rare that it is considered a freak occurrence.

Still, the parents' questions above are good ones and deserve thoughtful answers. These questions are the major motivation for this book. I want to answer all of them and more. To that end, this book will answer almost all the questions I have been asked by parents over the years. It will explain, in plain English, what mental disorders are and what treatments are available—with a focus on psychotropic drugs, as that is where most of the controversy is centered. I believe in the careful use of medication, but I am not blind to the controversies that exist and the many aspects of the mind that are still mysteries to all of us. With such mysteries come questions about treatments—that's only logical. The information in this book is based on long, hard, everyday clinical experience in the field treating young people. Differing points of view will be presented and the sensational fallacies pointed out. You will not come away from this book with absolute certainty about all aspects of giving children psychiatric medicine, but you will hopefully gain an appreciation of all the work that has gone into understanding children's problems and the enormous strides that have been made toward finding real solutions through the use of safe medications. While far short of miracle cures, psychotropic medications are safe and save lives, families, and futures.

Who Am I?

What qualifies me to write a book about young people taking psychotropic medication? I am a licensed psychiatrist specializing in children and adolescents and have been practicing in New York City for over thirty years. After medical school and an internal medicine internship, I studied adult psychiatry and then child and adolescent psychiatry in two successive residencies. I also studied psychoanalysis.

In my practice I have evaluated, treated, and prescribed medication for literally thousands of children and teenagers and have followed the progress of many of them over the course of many years. I have seen children in nearly all settings, including hospitals, outpatient public clinics, residences, foster agencies, and in private practice. I have written three books on the subject of children and teens and have appeared on hundreds of local and national television and radio shows. I have also supervised child and adolescent psychiatric residents and I teach mental health professionals from all fields.

As a result of my specialty, I have extensive experience prescribing all of the current psychotropic drugs and have treated children and teenagers with all the varied disorders listed in the diagnostic manuals. I have seen the therapeutic effects of medication when administered properly, the harmful effects when they are abused or prescribed incorrectly, and I have seen the side effects that do, very rarely, occur.

While I certainly don't believe that all children with mental disorders need medication, I strongly feel that some do. To withhold these important therapeutic agents can be harmful and, in some cases, tragic. I understand the anxiety that parents have about giving their children psychotropic drugs, and I have seen the devastation that can result in a child or teenager not getting the treatment they need. This is another reason why I'm writing this book. I have a deep sympathy for the children who suffer from mental problems and equal compassion for their parents. I respect the need for sound information, informed reassurance, and ongoing guidance during the time that a child is being treated.

CHAPTER ONE

YOUR QUESTIONS ANSWERED

What is a mental disorder? How do I know if my son has one?

Many people wonder when a child crosses the line between the normal variations in mood, behavior, and thinking that occur as they grow to having a more serious condition called a mental disorder. Since parents know their children better than anyone, they still make the best diagnosticians. Parents can reassure themselves if they get to know their particular child—their ways of relating and reacting to events, people and problems; their temperament or nature—while keeping in mind the incredibly wide normal variation in children. Armed with such specific knowledge about her child, a parent will know if a feeling, behavior, or thinking pattern seems unusual for that child. But even then we have to be careful and patient because as children and teenagers develop, they change, sometimes frequently, as a natural part of growing up. If this change is negative and doesn't show signs of going away, then it's time to take notice. The questions you should ask yourselves as parents are:

- Is my child not responding to our efforts to help him?
- Is her behavior interfering with her everyday life at school, with friends, with her siblings, with us?

- Is it affecting his personal activities like grooming, sleeping, and eating?
- Is the problem getting worse?

If you've answered yes to even one of these questions, then you should consider the possibility that your child may be suffering from a mental disorder.

Children and teenagers can suffer from a host of mental disorders, just like adults. Technically a mental disorder is defined as: "a clinically significant behavioral or psychological syndrome or pattern that occurs in an individual and that is associated with present distress (i.e., a painful symptom) or disability (i.e., impairment in one or more important areas of functioning) or with an increased risk of suffering death, pain, disability or an important loss of freedom." (Diagnostic and Statistical Manual of Mental Disorders, 4th Edition, DSM IV, American Psychiatric Association, 1994). These disorders are not just variations of normal development but are pretty well described syndromes.

The majority of young people with mental disorders suffer from some form of:

1. **Anxiety** such as school or other phobias, separation fears, panic disorder, obsessive-compulsive disorder, stress syndromes, and generalized anxiety (worrying too much).

2. **Disruptive Behavior Disorders** like attention deficit hyperactivity disorder, oppositional defiant disorder, and conduct disorder and:

3. **Mood Disorders** including depression and bipolar disorder.

In addition to those three major categories, we find young people suffering from:

- Substance abuse
- Psychoses (including schizophrenia)
- Autism
- Psychosomatic disorders
- Language and learning disorders
- Wetting and soiling
- Sleep disorders
- Gender identity disorder
- Eating disorders
- Tics
- Fire setting
- Stealing
- Tantrums
- Explosive anger
- Self-injurious behaviors (cutting, hair pulling)
- Pain syndromes
- Body dysmorphic disorder and hypochondriasis
- Selective mutism

There are also combinations of disorders. The severity of these mental disorders varies from mild to severe and incapacitating.

Why does my daughter have a mental disorder? Is it my fault?

It's natural to ask ourselves as parents, "What went wrong?" and, "Could I have prevented this from happening?" This is a difficult issue, as there is evidence that mental disorders usually stem from a combination of sources. The truth is no one really knows the exact cause of mental disorders. This complicated subject can be broken down as follows. There are at least four factors, two internal and two external, which contribute to some degree in the development of a mental disorder:

A. Internal Causes

1. **Genes**—There is evidence of some psychiatric problems running in families, but not as much as the media would have us believe.

2. **Neurotransmitter Chemicals**—These chemicals in our nervous system are concerned with the transmission of nervous impulses and have been implicated as being out of balance in the bodies of those with a mental disorder. This has never been proven, and no chemical imbalance has ever been shown to be a direct cause of a mental disorder despite many specialists saying and thinking so. These neurotransmitters are often identified as being the chemicals which psychotropic drugs act upon—"restore to balance"—but even the manufacturers of these drugs state that these are just hypotheses which have not been proven. Maybe some day we will know more about the details of these neurotransmitters and if and how they cause mental disorders, but for now we have to be content with knowing that many of them are treatable.

B. External Causes

1. **Severe Trauma**—Physical or sexual abuse, neglect, or other severe events such as losing one's family members are known to contribute to a higher rate of mental disorder, but interestingly, the majority of victims of these events don't necessarily develop a mental disorder.

2. **Parenting**—Parents and/or other significant caregivers influence a child's development, and while we do know that parents' ways often contribute to a child's problems, there is still not ample evidence to absolutely correlate a particular parenting style with the development of a specific disorder.

Despite our lack of complete understanding of what causes them, we do know that mental disorders are caused by some combination of internal and external factors. We will probably come to find that a genetic/biological/chemical predisposition makes a particular child more or less vulnerable to developing a disorder when exposed to some external trauma or parenting style. Research continues at a high rate and progress toward understanding the whys is growing.

Will the medication treat my son's symptoms, his disorder, or both?

Remember a mental disorder is a group of signs or symptoms. Psychotropic drugs treat those problems. But many psychiatrists—myself included—see these signs and symptoms as only part of the overall problem. Some feel these are like a fever—an indicator of an underlying and not so obvious condition. When our temperature goes up, maybe we have an infection somewhere which hasn't made itself known yet. So there is probably a great deal of truth to the idea that psychotropic drugs are treating the symptoms only. For biological psychiatrists—often those most recently trained—symptom focus and psychotropic drugs are the mainstay of the cure: fix the symptom and the problem is fixed. But for more psychoanalytically trained psychiatrists, there is much more to the story. We are just as interested in the underlying problems as we are in the patient's symptoms.

But what are those underlying problems? To believe in the concept *underlying* one has to believe in another concept: the unconscious mind—the belief that we have thoughts and feelings of which we are unaware. Freud's discovery of the unconscious mind entered mainstream psychiatry over a century ago. My clinical experience, as well as that of my thousands of colleagues who work everyday in the curious world of underlying issues, makes it clear that signs and symptoms have their origins deeper in the personality. What is their cause? In a nutshell, I believe that stresses in early life can lead to unresolved conflicts and anxiety. Many of us outgrow these difficulties as we mature. For others, the underlying tension leads to signs and symptoms which we call mental disorders. Which signs and symptoms we develop is based mostly on our genetic makeup. We can treat the symptoms very well with psychotropic medication, but it is almost always necessary to explore the underlying issues to free a person to develop to his full potential. That is why, paradoxically, a mental disorder can often lead to not only medication treatment but to an even more liberating therapy where underlying conditions can be clarified and cured. So like a fever treated with aspirin that leads to our getting antibiotics for a strep throat, a psychiatric symptom can often lead to medication and a more thorough cure. Thus, I almost never prescribe medication without a recommendation for psychotherapy as well. But for many children and teenagers, the symptoms are so bad that therapy can't even take place until medication brings some relief.

In summary, the use of medication treats symptoms, which are usually the expression of deeper issues that must be overcome as well for someone to get better and grow toward a full life. All this is why I believe that the use of medication is mostly helpful to symptom relief—no small accomplishment—and will often give a child enough of a reprieve from her symptoms to gain from other therapies, ranging from talk therapy to special educational settings, resulting in growth and maturation for the child and family.

I've heard there's an increase in prescribing medication to children. Why?

The use of child and adolescent psychotropic drugs started about seventy years ago with the use of stimulants to treat hyperactive children. As time passed, several trends came together into making the use of the many modern psychotropic drugs so common:

The pharmaceutical industry has been doing more and more research leading to the production of many compounds found useful for treating mental disorders. Not only were the number of stimulants increased, but the manufacture and use of many antidepressants, antipsychotic medications, and mood stabilizing compounds flourished in the last thirty years and continues today.

Drug companies started aggressive marketing of these compounds.

At the same time that drug manufacturers increased their interest in these drugs, the psychiatric profession has also turned to refining diagnostic criteria for child and adolescent disorders. The number of conditions has increased, diagnostic manuals continue to grow, and special screening tests and interest in diagnosing young people flourishes. This shift to diagnosing and categorizing fits neatly into the use of medication tailored to various symptom pictures.

There has been a shift in American psychiatry in general toward diagnosis and the search for a biological causation for illnesses, away from more traditional psychoanalytic views (this has been called the "remedicalization of psychiatry" and what some feel is a return to 19th century ideas where categorization reigned). As a result, there has been an increase of biological research and various medical diagnostic procedures (brain scans and biochemical research, for instance) which still have as yet to show much everyday clinical significance.

The increasing pressure of insurance companies to want to cut face-to-face therapy sessions in favor of quicker medication management sessions.

The general increase in preference for quick medication cures for all illnesses and thus a general increase in prescribing for all diseases in this country.

As the trend toward increased prescribing has continued there have been backlashes all around, including criticism of the vagueness and inaccuracy of diagnosing rapidly changing young people. It is true that there is little known about the effects of these drugs on future development. Side effects have also been a cause of increased worry. There have been false reports of high numbers of deaths from psychotropic medication. Some have worried that these drugs actually make children worse. Finally, there has always been the concern that psychotropic drug companies rarely test these compounds on children, and so the drugs are often prescribed in an "off label" fashion by physicians—a frequent phenomenon in all fields of medicine.

Many of the arguments against increased prescribing have taken on somewhat of a social movement character, even enlisting popular celebrities like Tom Cruise to take up the cause. The Internet has been flooded with fantastic tales of horror associated with medication use alongside more rational questioning of the trend.

But none of this has really lessened the use of psychotropic medication until recently when there was great concern about the use of one type of antidepressant (SSRI) causing increased suicidality in young people under twenty-five years old. There was a great cutback in its use which, unfortunately, led to a dramatic decrease in diagnosing of depression and an increase in suicidality in teenagers. Ultimately, reexamination of the original data has left doubts as to the accuracy of the prior conclusions (fortunately, the suicide rate has dropped off again as antidepressant prescribing has gone back up).

So there is little evidence that psychotropic drug use will decrease in the foreseeable future. Important questions remain; questions that each parent has to weigh with their prescribing professional. Parents deserve accurate information, and medication use should be a collaborative venture between families and doctors.

Can our pediatrician prescribe psychotropic medication for my daughter?

In the United States, doctors without special psychiatric training write the great majority of prescriptions for psychotropic medications. Although it is difficult to quantify, it appears that psychiatrists write only about 20–25 percent. Although it would be preferable to have all of these prescriptions written by a psychiatrist, with children and teenagers it is even more important. Why? Because the practice of prescribing these specialized medications requires specific knowledge of children and teenagers that is only gained by those who have completed special training in child and adolescent psychiatry in approved residency programs.

A general (adult) psychiatrist goes to medical school and then completes post graduate specialty training of four years of general psychiatry. A child and adolescent psychiatrist then goes on for an additional two years. Thus he receives training in general psychiatry first and then specialized training in child and adult psychiatry.

In a child and adolescent residency, we learn about the details of child/teenage/family development in all areas: biological, neurological, educational, psychological, emotional, and physical realms. We learn about the field of pediatrics and are able to integrate physical illness and its affects into our diagnostic and treatment expertise. We have detailed exposure to the diagnosis of all the mental disorders that occur in the formative years, both in outpatient and hospital settings. We study feelings, behaviors, and thinking patterns. In addition, we get exposure to all the various modes of therapeutic intervention including individual, family, and group talk therapy.

In a child and adolescent psychiatry residency, we scrutinize the use of psychotropic drugs for the many disorders of childhood and teenagers. We study not only the helping effects of medications but the side effects, the use of multiple medications, the emotional repercussions of taking medication on the child and family, and the introduction of medication to school personnel when necessary. Most importantly, we learn about the unique metabolism of medication by young people.

Only about eight thousand doctors are trained in child and adolescent psychiatry in the United States. This is a small amount and the field is considered very understaffed. Because of this, it will not always be possible to see a trained child and adolescent psychiatrist, especially if you live in a rural area. Pediatricians, clinic nurse practitioners, and general psychiatrists are the other major prescribing groups for child and adolescent psychotropics and although the great majority have skill in this area, it is best to find out how much experience they have with young people in particular. You can simply ask your doctor directly about their education, continuing education, and of course, direct patient care experience. Additionally you can search the Internet, consult with local mental health associations, and with the referring person (pediatrician) to learn more about the doctor in question.

Is it true that most psychotropic drugs are not approved for use in young people?

In the United States the Federal Drug Administration (FDA) approves a drug for use. The process is lengthy and expensive. A typical drug is usually first tested in the laboratory, then in animal trials, and then in several phases of human testing. The FDA is looking for effectiveness and safety.

After the drug is approved, prescribing doctors are free to use it not only for people with the disease for which approval was given, and not only for the age group that was tested, but for anyone the medical community deems might benefit from the drug's use. Prescribing for people of different ages and those with different conditions is called off-label prescribing. Believe it or not, it is estimated that over half of all prescribing of the many billions of dollars of drugs each year in all medical specialties is off label. And in psychiatry, and especially child and adolescent psychiatry, the percentage is estimated to be anywhere between 55–85 percent.

The reason for such high numbers of off-label prescribing is that the arduous process of getting approval could not possibly cover all uses and age groups. Testing and getting approval to use all drugs for all reasonable conditions and uses would make it practically impossible to treat people who need medicines since it would take extra decades and many extra billions of dollars to cover everyone who would need approval. The wisdom and practicality of medical professionals is relied upon for making decisions based on experience. Off-label prescribing is legal and supported by the courts and medical associations.

In child and adolescent psychiatry, the majority of the drug prescribing is done off-label. Few medications are approved for young people, but making these valuable medications unavailable because drug companies have not tested them for all conditions and populations would cause a lot of prolonged suffering and even deaths. This is the case for hundreds of drugs, not just psychotropics. Studies have been coming out showing the helpfulness of psychotropic medication in young people and hopefully science and research will continue to catch up with clinical reality.

All in all, there are about ninety common psychotropic medications in common use today. The highest rate of approved drugs for use in children is in the area of stimulants used for ADHD. In that category 100 percent of the drugs are approved for young people. In the antidepressant category, there are about thirty compounds altogether, seven of which are approved for use in children. In the antipsychotic category (most of these drugs are used for behavior control), there are fewer than twenty compounds with seven approved for children. There are no officially approved drugs for the treatment of anxiety in children and teens, and for mood stabilization (bipolar children) six medications are approved, mainly for teenagers only.

So, yes, child and adolescent psychiatrists routinely prescribe off label, but we know that what we are prescribing works. Although there have been outcries against any off-label drug use because of possible dangers, the other side of the argument is that millions of people would be hurt if medication were withheld. When it comes to children, the outcry is even louder since the vulnerability is assumed to be greater with a younger and more physically and mentally immature population. But despite the many Internet tales of children being harmed by off-label prescribing, there are few reports in professional journals of its particular danger.

Can these medications harm my son? I've heard that kids have died from taking them.

Almost any medication prescribed for any condition carries some risk of unwanted side effects. In fact, even everyday medications like aspirin, antihistamines, and other common remedies have dangers—albeit rare. Despite what we hear, see and read, psychotropic drugs rarely cause serious side effects. When they do, however, they can be bothersome and sometimes lead to the psychiatrist having to stop them. These side effects will be covered later in this book as we discuss particular drugs.

But let's talk about safety, an issue that concerns everyone, especially when it comes to our children. To my knowledge, psychotropic drugs, when taken correctly and monitored by a qualified child and adolescent psychiatrist, are very safe. I have never witnessed a death or ever heard of a case of death caused by psychotropic drugs. I have read innumerable articles about this subject, continuously monitor the professional literature, and confer with colleagues—and still no reports have shown up. There has been concern about certain ADHD drugs causing cardiac death but this has never been proven. There is suspicion that some heart problems might occur in children who have pre-existing heart conditions. Also there has been some concern about antipsychotic medications and some antidepressants causing heart rhythm disturbances which might cause death, in theory, but no bona fide cases have been reported. There have been serious warnings about some antidepressant drugs indirectly causing death by increasing suicidal behavior—this resulted in the "Black Box warning"—which in turn led to a drastic decrease in the prescription of these medications to young people. But the validity of the original studies is questionable, and unfortunately we saw a great rise in suicide directly attributable to this change in prescribing habits. There is also some concern about the combining of certain psychotropic medications causing death, but autopsy studies in these very rare cases revealed pre-existing cardiac problems. Very recently a study was published which hinted about a possible connection between ADHD medication and sudden death, but that one study was very small and resulted in widespread doubt as to its validity and meaning.

So all in all, side effects are usually easily dealt with and fatalities from taking psychotropic drugs are either non-existent or so rare and unreported that I think we can safely assume that this is not a serious danger. But there is a danger in taking psychotropic drugs in combination with other types of drugs or even, in rare cases, with other psychotropics that might cause potentially lethal conditions. But that is no different than any drug combination. That is why it is so crucial that parents let any prescribing physician know of any medications that a child is taking—including alternative remedies—and also that the doctor know of any use of illegal substances, even alcohol, which in combination with psychotropics can be dangerous.

It is also crucial that a full medical history be given to the prescribing physician since giving certain psychotropic medication to a child with a medical condition can be very dangerous, such as administering medication which might have a tendency to cause seizures to a child with epilepsy, or giving ADHD medication to a child with certain heart conditions.

How do we know there aren't long term negative effects of the medications?

Naturally, parents worry about long-term negative effects of psychotropic medication on children. We have very little data since most of the psychotropic drug explosion has been relatively recent and not enough time has passed to see any long-term effects on the brain or development in general. But even for very common psychotropic drugs like Ritalin, which has been used for fifty years, there has been no evidence that there are long-term dangers. At this time there is no documented reason to worry about psychotropic drugs causing death or long-term damage to our children. While some of the side effects like drowsiness, mood changes, or other symptoms can affect our children, these are easily recognized and treated if the medication is being monitored correctly. Even for drugs that have been used for fifty years there is no evidence of long-term damage to children except for relatively minor issues like a very small height diminution in children who have taken some of the ADHD medications—and even in this case it is not known if the decrease lasts into adulthood.

Lastly, there are always the newspaper headlines about famous or not so famous people dying from psychotropic drugs. This is very different from dying from proper prescribing. In these cases there is usually an overdose of the drug, either intentionally or otherwise, a combination of drugs, or an interaction with illicit drugs or alcohol.

How do these drugs work?

If the truth be known, we really don't know how these psychotropic drugs work in people. Most of the articles published in psychiatric journals talk about mechanisms of action of these compounds. There is exhaustive discussion of the chemistry of the compounds and where specifically in the brain they do their business. But even the manufacturers of the medications mention that there is only a presumption of how they work—not any definite knowledge. It isn't really that surprising in light of the enormous complexity of human beings, especially in the area of our emotions, thoughts, and behavior. To be able to pinpoint the specific target when our brains are so infinitely complex and full of billions of nerve cells and chemicals is almost impossible to imagine. It is mere reductionism and simplicity that tempts people to say that the exact mechanisms of action are known. What we do know is that the drugs work.

Most of the theories about the action of these medications have to do with chemical effects. This is why chemical imbalances are often hypothesized as being the cause of mental disorders. In fact, there is no known chemical imbalance proven yet. Yet nearly everyone involved in the billions of dollars of research writes about these drugs affecting various chemicals in the brain. The most common theory is that chemicals called neurotransmitters act in the synapses, the spaces between nerve connections. Various neurotransmitters are said to be produced by a nerve cell on one side of a synapse and travel across the synapse to the other nerve cell. By increasing or decreasing the concentration of the transmitter in these spaces, these drugs supposedly exert their effects. We hear mostly about the neurotransmitters serotonin, dopamine, and norepinepherine. The models seem straightforward and the diagrams used seem so logical that it is inviting to believe that this has all been proven, but no such luck. While there are strong hints about these chemical theories, there is no proof yet. In fact, there are some studies that show opposite effects from similar drugs, and the same effects from drugs which are supposed to work differently. For example, most of us have heard that if we increase the availability of serotonin at a synapse then depressed patients will get better, and those drugs that supposedly do that help with major depression. But other drugs which are said to decrease available serotonin also help with depression. Another interesting example of some of the confusion is that well-known electroconvulsive therapy helps some people with depression. It causes a massive electrical brain seizure but we have no idea how it works. Some people have even gone as far as saying that any jolt we give to the chemicals in the nervous system might be enough to help with mental suffering.

Should we withhold these medications because science has not caught up with clinical experience? I think that would be wrong. Science may well catch up, and in the meantime these drugs help children and teenagers. An enormous amount of research continues to be done, and doctors are always watching and recording adverse effects, making for an excellent safety profile.

Simply said: Don't believe everything you're told about how all these medications work, but do believe that they work pretty well. As a rule of thumb, choose medications that have had decent clinical trials and have been approved by the FDA. And most of all, don't feel that your child has some chemical imbalance, but understand that he might benefit from a chemical intervention combined with other measures.

The doctor said my daughter might need to take more than one drug. Isn't that dangerous?

Up to one third of adults who take psychotropic medication take more than one—this is called polypharmacy. This happens with young people, too. There are many different reasons for this which I'll explain below. Don't be surprised if your child's psychiatrist suggests a combination of drug therapies.

In this event, there are concerns and the prescriber should take great care in explaining them. When taking more than one drug, there is an increased possibility of side effects, problematic adverse reactions, and interactions amongst the drugs. There is also a good chance that you'll be spending more money.

Doctors will prescribe more than one drug for several reasons. We might introduce a new drug at the same time the patient is withdrawing from one that did not work; or try to get a better response—augmentation—by adding new drugs; or treat symptoms from different disorders which require different medications. Multiple mental conditions are quite common and this is called comorbidity. Psychiatric disorders that are often comorbid with others include but are not limited to: the behavior disorders (ADHD, oppositional defiant disorder, conduct disorder), bipolar disorder, obsessive compulsive disorder, tic syndromes, depression and anxiety, autism, and intermittent explosive disorder. The rule is to try to treat the most serious first and then tend to the less severe. So for instance, if severe ADHD is first treated with Ritalin we might also see a long-term depression which needs treatment later on.

We know that it is always best to start with one psychotropic medication for any psychiatric condition. But sometimes there is either a weak or even no response. At that point the psychiatrist has several choices. Best would be to try another drug, possibly one from the first class of drugs or from a different class. But the first drug must be tapered, and most of the time the second is started during the tapering of the first. This is done carefully and slowly. At this point we have entered the realm of temporary polypharmacy. Another common situation is when two disabling symptoms exist and two drugs are needed, for example a severe depression with crippling anxiety. Then starting simultaneously with an antidepressant and adding a tranquilizer is common. Children with bipolar disorder often need a mood stabilizer as well as an antipsychotic medication as both an enhancer and to control out-of-control behavior or mania. Many people need sleeping medication while their primary psychotropic medication takes time to work and sleep is still disturbed.

Whatever the situation, your prescriber should sit down with you and explain to you the reasons for multiple medications; the specific symptoms he is treating and why; the possible adverse effects; how long each medication should take to work; and, of course, a reliable and regular plan for monitoring the situation. And be certain to let the prescriber know of any other medications your child might be taking, including over the counter medications and alternative remedies.

In summary: usually only one drug will be introduced to start. If it does not work well then another should be tried while the first gets tapered. If there is still a problem, then additional medication should be tried slowly, and your doctor should explain fully the risks and benefits. Don't panic when you hear, "More than one medication is needed." It is common practice and quite safe. I do it regularly and rarely encounter a problem.

Will my son have to take medication for the rest of his life?

This question is very common and sensible. I think that often what is behind the question is another: "How impaired is my child, and is there any hope?" In some way the answer to how long might give a parent some indication as to how bad things really are. But let's assume that the question is just what it is.

Most of the time there is no definite answer to this important question. Unlike some medical conditions which might necessitate lifelong therapy like diabetes, adult heart disease, and the like, with children and mental disorders things are much more fluid, and actually, more hopeful.

Although all of us can grow emotionally until the day we die, the younger we are, the more likely that the rapid growth process of youth, the degree of flexibility, and the possibility of important environmental influences improving will all contribute toward improvement of a young person's problems. Additionally, the use of psychotropic medication is usually only a part of the therapeutic process for any particular child, so it will help the child benefit from talk therapy, adjustments in your parenting style, and classroom improvements. Thus the medication doesn't only make your child feel better, it will also give him the chance to benefit better from other therapies. That is a major reason we don't really know at first how long the medication might have to be prescribed.

We also don't know how a particular child will react to a given medication. There might be no response to the first medication and several might have to be prescribed to find just the right one. Or there might be side effects that necessitate a change. And, as I mentioned above, it might be necessary to combine more than one medication to get the desired effect.

Assuming there is success, as there usually is, we can then ask how long the treatment should last. In general, I prefer that the child stay on the medication long enough to experience a good deal of time free of troubling and painful symptoms—measured in months at a minimum. It is startling to see the relief a child experiences when he is treated for ADHD and is finally able to concentrate and learn. Or to see a child emerge from a state of chronic despair and lack of enjoyment due to depression. Or to watch a severely behavior-disordered child finally be able to be a good student and stop getting suspended or punished. This is all possible when children are treated with the right medication. We see it every day: children who get better, feel better, experience hope, and stop feeling alienated. It is good that they feel like that for a while, if for no other reason than to know that it is possible. If, at the same time, the parents can change their ways, conflicts get resolved, physical and mental maturing take place, people in the schools stop labeling the child, friendships blossom, and the child feels more integrated into society, then the medication has helped a great deal. Add in talk therapy, making it more possible to attend to issues, and the benefit of medication becomes even clearer.

In general, the use of medication is measured in months and maybe even years, but certainly not in weeks as many parents hope. For a small minority of children with very severe conditions like psychosis, it might even be necessary to plan on an indefinite amount of time. Although we all wish for quick miracle cures, there aren't any yet. Educating yourself through reliable sources, staying patient, listening to professional guidance, having faith in your doctor about his monitoring any dangers, and trusting in the inherent growth potential of your child will make the wait to stop the medication more tolerable.

Later on, when we discuss particular medications, we will review time courses of medication in more detail. But keep in mind we can never promise a definite timetable; we can only give a good hunch. Remember, too, that the more experience we have treating youngsters with similar conditions, the better our hunches will be.

What happens to kids who don't take the recommended medication?

This question is one that is not so easy to answer as there are not enough long-term studies of every mental disorder to be definitive about outcomes. In other words, the natural history of mental disorders has not been fully researched.

But we do know enough to make some general comments. The ability to overcome anxiety and other problems increases with age if the environment is not so severe as to short circuit that process. Going through puberty often has an ameliorative effect for many children who have a mental disorder. And children who are living in homes where there are obvious external stressors do well enough without medication if the problems are solved in some way. For example, if a child suffers from a ongoing severe stress syndrome like child abuse, then this child will probably not get better—in fact, he will probably get worse over time. On the other hand, even a severely symptomatic child who is suffering from a tumultuous divorce struggle will often get better after things settle down. In that case I would probably not suggest medication at first but instead try to help the parents resolve their differences. So, in general, when there are obvious mild to moderate stressors causing a disorder which eventually cease (i.e. change of neighborhoods, loss of a pet), the child stands a pretty good chance of remitting, with patience and some form of advice/counseling probably doing the trick. The presence of severe events (abuse, death of a parent) even if one time still require some form of intervention. Independent of the type or duration of a stressor though whenever there is severe symptomology like suicidal ideas, depression interfering with functioning in everyday activities, or violence, for example, then a medication prescription is probably indicated.

There are many other problems that require therapeutic intervention with medication. These are syndromes that might not get better or even get worse and have wider ramifications if untreated. For example, the well-known attention deficit syndrome, if untreated, often leads to chronic low self-esteem, interpersonal problems, educational failure, teenage substance abuse, alienation, isolation, family problems, and stigmatization. Medication used in the early years could help prevent many of these secondary manifestations of the syndrome, as well as the symptoms of the disorder itself. Depression is another problem that often requires medication. Although major depression often has a limited life if untreated, there are enough times that medication will hasten recovery and help avoid school failure, interpersonal deterioration, and suicide. In some young people, their aggression is so out of control that they can in fact end up hurting someone, getting arrested, and being placed out of the house without proper medication. Severely disturbed children suffering from a psychosis or pervasive development disorder suffer greatly and often find it impossible to stay in the house without the use of medication.

Thus, while many children outgrow their difficulties without the use of medication, there are those whose problems will get worse if not treated with medication. But it should be remembered that the ideal treatment for almost any child is some form of talk therapy along with medication. It is a rare child whom I will medicate who is also not in some form of therapy.

How much research should I do when the doctor prescribes medication for my child?

It is natural for a parent to worry when a medication is prescribed for their developing child. That's why it is very important that the prescribing psychiatrist takes time to discuss all aspects of medication at the time of prescribing and on an ongoing basis. Goals of treatment, as well as common side effects, should be explained. Questions should be fielded cooperatively. Informed consent should be routine.

But even after that, many parents who live in our information age still have worries and further questions. They often turn to written material they find on the pharmacy drug sheet or the Internet.

In theory, this is a good idea, but unfortunately it often leaves parents scared as they read highly technical data and sometimes even plainly wrong information. I often get urgent calls from parents after they read of a particular side effect which was not discussed, not realizing that the side effect is extremely rare to the point of clinical insignificance and thus was not discussed in our meeting. So many side effects are listed for every drug that if they were all believed to be serious or common many people would take nothing—not even aspirin. The experience and wisdom of the prescriber should help you weigh the benefits and risks of a drug for your child. Many patients call me with these questions, and I usually say that a particular effect is true but rare and should be put aside compared to the benefits of the prescribed drug. Nothing substitutes for clinical experience and the doctor's ability to understand and evaluate what is meant by the written word.

The one caveat I have for parents who use the Internet to research medication is that there is often fallacious material posted by overemotional parents or others who frankly misstate facts. The Internet is full of false claims as to the dangers of medications. Dangers are often made up, reported out of context, exaggerated, distorted, and discussed from a one-sided point of view. The websites that some parents tend to stumble across are often written by nonprofessionals and testimonials are usually filled with generalizations, distorted anecdotes, or even false rumors having little to do with proper prescribing. I spend a great deal of time explaining to concerned parents how to interpret something they have read into a less anxious context and directing them to the more reliable websites or other sources of correct information. This is part of the art of prescribing medication. And doctors must remain patient, as these calls are from worried parents who want the best for their children.

Should medication be tried immediately?

Sometimes it is quite evident from the beginning that medication will be needed right away. Some examples would be for an out-of-control child who is so violent that the lives of others and the child herself are in jeopardy. This often happens when a child becomes psychotic, explosive, or even acutely intoxicated. Another time might be when a depressed child has become so hopeless that suicide has become the only option she can consider. Other times that the psychiatrist will consider medication right off the bat are:

- When a parent reports that all other interventions have failed to ameliorate the condition
- There has been ongoing individual or family therapy
- Intense behavioral interventions by multiple caregivers such as at school or special programs has failed
- The family is so disrupted that they are ready to send the child away if there is no immediate help
- If the parents are so unavailable due to various reasons that they cannot help in a treatment plan, and the child is worsening like in an addictive family, a rancorous battling family, or when someone is very ill
- When it is quite clear that the child has such a mental impairment that any form of verbal therapy will not help, and there are worsening symptoms such as in children with developmental problems which impair social interaction
- Bedwetting that has been going on to the point of such shame and embarrassment that social life is severely impaired
- When a child has begun to lose touch with reality in the form of hearing voices, seeing things, and thinking and acting in bizarre fashion
- When a child becomes acutely manic to the point of severe social and psychological disintegration

Barring these extreme examples, using medication is generally not considered until some other form of therapy has been tried. But this is easier said than done. Many places have a great shortage of trained therapists with experience with young people. Thus the psychiatrist will have few referral sources.

I always try to set up some form of what we call psychological intervention preceding the use of medication. For people with mental disorders, talk therapy of some sort is still the gold standard of intervention, be it individual, group, family, parent/child, psychodynamic (looking at underlying causes), or behavioral. School intervention can also be helpful, so consulting with teachers and guidance counselors is important. Sometimes a change of classrooms, remediation, or some form of time out or rest period goes a long way to ameliorating problems. Pediatricians should always be involved to be sure of physical well being and often blood tests will be ordered just to be sure there is no physical ailment expressing itself through a mental condition. Occasionally calling in other family members, grandma and grandpa for example, to help out, can relieve a lot of trouble. Or even having one person leave the house for a while—an abusive spouse, for instance—might lead to calmness. Joining after school activities, especially ones geared to children with particular issues, can often help as well.

If the problem remains after an adequate trial, the prescribing psychiatrist often turns to medication. Medication isn't viewed as a cure, but rather as an adjunct to all the other help being offered. A child who feels a bit better can participate more in his own treatment than one so impaired that his feelings of hopelessness interfere with getting the help needed.

What's involved in a psychiatric evaluation of my youngster?

At some point you might find it necessary to get a psychiatric evaluation for your child. The suggestion might come from a teacher, a therapist, or even from yourself. You can usually find a child and adolescent psychiatrist from your pediatrician, school personnel, clergy, or very often from a friend whose child has also gotten help. If all else fails, a call to your local mental health association or your local hospital will lead you in the right direction

You will probably call the doctor and explain briefly why you are calling. Quite often, after hearing a story, I suggest that people wait a while, especially if I feel that what is being described is minor or possibly a passing developmental phenomenon which will soon be outgrown. I suggest calling me in several weeks in these cases to report in. Sometimes a doctor cannot ascertain enough from an initial phone call, and you will be asked to come in. At other times it is clear from the outset that the parents want an in-person consultation, or I feel that one is needed.

If a consultation seems necessary, the psychiatrist usually sees the parent(s) before seeing the child unless an adolescent over the age of about thirteen years old needs help. In the latter case, it is best to see the teenager first to establish trust and to emphasize the fact that that there will be respect of the teenager's privacy and boundaries with her parents. In most cases the teen's parents are seen later, preferably in the presence of their youngster.

During the initial sessions with the psychiatrist you will probably be asked many questions about why you are seeking consultation. The doctor will ask about problems with behavior, moods, learning, thinking, family relations, and physical health. What medications are being taken? Are there unusual habits, isolation, anger, anxiety, regression to immature behaviors, interpersonal difficulties, behavioral problems at home or school, or self-destructive behavior? Is your child getting worse or better? Has there been a recent fast upsurge of dangerous behavior? Is there an emergency brewing? Have there been major life changes? Death? Illness? A move? A separation? New school? Financial problems? A change in lifestyle? You will be asked about a timeline of the development of the problem, as well as ways you have tried to help. You will be asked about your own problems, the family constellation, and other siblings who might have troubles. You will be asked about your marriage, divorce, separation, step-parenting, and other pertinent issues. A history will be taken about the pregnancy, birth, early developmental milestones, and all aspects of your child's life including, but not limited to, family functioning, friends, school activities, after school activities, and sleeping and eating habits as well as your child's overall temperament, personality, and physical health. You will be asked about your attitudes about discipline. What's the family atmosphere like? Is it a loud but loving house? Is there always anger? Is it a quiet overly controlled atmosphere? Is there substance abuse in the house? Is there domestic violence or abuse of the child? Have there been recent stressors, family upheaval, illness in a family member, or other triggers? A history of any previous therapies, medications past and present, as well as possible hospitalizations will be asked for.

By the end of what might seem an exhaustive questioning period, the psychiatrist will have a pretty good idea about the child who is the focus of the consultation request as well as many other members of the family.

At this point you might simply get reassurance that the problem seems minor, if not just a passing phase, and be given some informed advice to help clear the road of your child's development. Maybe a different form of discipline, an understanding of your child's anger as a messenger of underlying distress, change of school, different bedtime ritual or time, a new family activity, or some other such intervention. You will be asked to call back and give the doctor a follow up.

At other times the psychiatrist will decide that it is necessary to see the child.

How do I tell my daughter I'm taking her to a psychiatrist?

I usually instruct parents to tell their child that they have been concerned about some issue, to name it, and then say they have spoken to a doctor who talks to children about such issues and that an appointment has been made. A good rule of thumb is to give the child enough notice in days for each year of age (for teenagers once or twice is enough). So for a six-year-old I would advise telling her each day for six days and giving a little reminder of the appointment with the talking doctor. For most children, that will suffice. For more anxious children, it might be necessary to describe me and the office, and maybe emphasize that there are no physical interventions like needles and that you will even come in the room with the child if necessary. But for the most part, it is better to downplay the appointment so fears won't build in anticipation. For example: "Joey, we made an appointment with Dr. Paul who talks to kids about school behavior. You can talk to him about what some of the teachers have been saying to you." At no time should the visit to a doctor be presented as punishment, as a last ditch effort because you "can't take it anymore," or for any reason other than to make your child feel better.

When you come to the office, you will usually be greeted by the doctor. In most cases, the child will be invited to come in on his own. If this proves impossible, I usually invite parents in, at least for the beginning of the session. Sometimes the parent(s) have to stay the whole time if there is high anxiety, but for the most part the parent can wait nearby in the waiting room after a short period of time.

The interview with the child is preferably conducted by simply speaking to the child. Believe it or not, most children liked being talked to as adults in the "adult seat" instead of being pulled into a playroom and bombarded with toys which in many cases serve as distractions. Some children who have difficulty conversing for whatever reason: age, anxiety, or language disorders, for example, will need the introduction of very limited aids such as drawing, writing, puppets, balls, dolls, etc., but I try to avoid elaborate games, exercise devices, cards, transformers, and the like.

I usually introduce myself as a doctor who speaks to children about worries, problems, nervousness, or school/family problems. I ask why he is here. In most cases I hear a response that shows that the child knows there is a problem. We explore the problem in as much detail as possible. After exhausting the presenting problem, I do an inventory interview in which I ask about other areas. For example, if the problem was behavior in school, I go over friendships, family life, hobbies, dreams, daydreams, physical problems, moods etc. In other words, I try to cover all the important areas of a child's life by the end of the interview: home, school (behavior and academics), after school activities, interpersonal relations, and body issues and self-image. It is often necessary to have an additional interview with the child to complete all of the above.

In such an interview, not only is information gathered, but the psychiatrist is also evaluating physical health, coordination, hearing, language and speech skills, eye contact, frustration tolerance, motor activity, relatedness, neurological issues, evidence of mood disturbances, and/or psychotic symptoms like false beliefs or hallucinations, temperament, degree of alertness, intelligence, suicidal or homicidal/violent trends, academic skills, expressivity, resilience, ability to cope with problems, sense of humor, and overall adjustment.

After seeing the child, I might ask to see the whole family together, especially if family issues are the focus of the problem. It can be enormously helpful to see how people communicate with each other.

After all of the questions and interviews, the psychiatrist formulates what the problem is. This process goes further than assigning the child a diagnosis from the manual. It offers a broader appreciation of the child's development, the family integrity, the school/ friend environment, and finally where things might be going wrong and a plan to get things back on track.

I then have a talk with the parents to present what I have tentatively found and what comes next. All in all, a child psychiatric evaluation can take up to four or five separate interviews. With teenagers it might be a bit less. By the time you leave the last interview, you should have a pretty good idea of what the psychiatrist thinks is the problem, the child and family's strengths, and if further diagnostic testing is needed. For instance: are psychological/learning/language evaluations needed; is a neurological evaluation necessary; should you talk with the pediatrician or teacher/tutor?

Lastly, a tentative treatment plan is made which should include the type of therapy that might be needed, including some form of talk/verbal therapy and possibly medication. You will have many questions, and there should be time allowed for this and further contact by telephone for questions which might enter your mind later. It should be kept in mind that you as a parent will always be involved in any form of treatment. After all, the goal is helping the child get on track in his environment, not in my office. From the beginning, the psychiatrist should be picturing the end of treatment and working toward that goal. Not only will you be involved in the treatment, but sometimes a recommendation might be made for you to get your own counseling or treatment, as any help and support you get and any progress you make in your life will reflect on your child as well.

CHAPTER TWO

WHAT YOU'LL NEED TO KNOW BEFORE STARTING YOUR CHILD ON MEDICATION

If you have been told that your child would benefit from taking medication, the following guide will help.

1. Have your doctor explain your child's diagnosis in as much detail as possible. Is there a known cause for the difficulty? What course might the disorder take if not treated? For example, if a child with ADHD doesn't get treatment, the chance of substance abuse increases as the teenage years approach. Teenagers not treated for depression have an increased suicide risk. What positive effects of the medication will the psychiatrist be looking for? How long should it take? What will he will do if it doesn't work? While there is no medication which totally cures everything, your child's prescription should target specific symptoms.

2. Make sure your child gets other forms of treatment along with medication. What does your doctor recommend? Individual talk therapy? Special school interventions? Behavioral therapy? Family counseling? Be wary of the practitioner who simply gives you a pill and wishes you good luck.

3. Make sure your child is physically healthy. If not, then the prescribing psychiatrist needs to be familiar with any medical condition. To this end, the doctor should take a detailed medical history of your child. In addition, I like to see a report of a recent physical examination from the child's pediatrician. I also suggest a routine blood screening including a complete blood count, a routine metabolic screening, and also a routine twelve lead electrocardiogram in most cases. The blood tests and EKG will not only give signs of present conditions but will serve as baseline readings. Some medications affect blood tests and the EKG, and if we don't have a baseline it will be difficult to know if future abnormal readings are caused by a medication or were always present.

4. Have a clear understanding of the medication's side effects. Most side effects are fleeting and mild and don't interfere much in your child's life in any way, but they can be specific depending on the medication. You should know what they are so you don't get worried. Serious or long lasting side effects for child and teenage psychotropic drugs are rare, but again, you should be told of the signs. If you read information from the internet, be careful about the websites you choose (see below). Don't jump to the conclusion that information you find online is more accurate than your psychiatrist's years of clinical prescribing experience.

5. Make sure your child's doctor, or a covering professional, is available twenty-four hours a day, 365 days a year, for any concerns you have about your child. Anything less is unacceptable.

6. Understand why the great majority of psychotropic medications given to young people are off label, which means

they haven't been specially approved for use by children (see above). You will want to ask your prescribing psychiatrist what his particular experience is with the medication as well as what studies have shown about its use in children and teenagers.

7. Find out from your doctor what time of day and how to give your child the medication—with meals, all pills at once, full or empty stomach? Although many pharmacies now include a written summary of various aspects of the drug, follow the prescriber's recommendations over those of the pharmacy. Call the doctor if there is a difference.

8. Determine what the medication will cost. Are there ways to cut the cost? Your pharmacist is the best source for that information. Cost alone should never force a decision as to choice of medication. Sometimes insurance companies make it difficult to get medication. Be persistent and get help from your psychiatrist to be sure your child gets exactly what the doctor ordered: generic or brand, the correct quantity, and refills if possible.

9. Ask if there is a difference between generic and brand name drugs. I have not seen much of a difference between their effectiveness. Generic is usually okay. Some patients demand brand name medications and I go along with it, but with the caveat that these will cost more money with little research showing a beneficial effect.

10. Tell your child's doctor about any other medications, supplements, or home remedies your child is receiving to be sure there are no adverse interactions with the prescribed

medication. Remember even natural remedies can cause interaction problems.

11. Never compare dosages in milligrams between medications; they all differ and cannot be compared because of potency differences in the manufacturing process. Thus one milligram of one medication might equal in efficacy ten milligrams of another. For example, I recently had to explain to a patient that the new medication I was giving was measured in one half to two milligrams dosages and was replacing one that measured about thirty milligrams. It was simply another compound whose potency was measured differently.

12. Be prepared for your child's doctor to recommend more than one medication (see above). This use of multiple medications has become more common, as it sometimes gives better results. There are, however, risks to this practice which your doctor will need to explain. Risks include medication interaction, increased side effects, as well as decreased compliance because of the difficulty some patients have with multiple prescriptions. Always find out why your doctor is prescribing multiple medications and ask specific questions about the benefits and risks of such prescribing.

13. Always trust yourself and all the knowledge you have about your child. No one knows her better than you and thus your observations of side effects, therapeutic effects, and overall well-being are the most valuable. Don't be intimidated. Call your psychiatrist with any concerns.

CHAPTER THREE

STIMULANT MEDICATIONS: WHEN YOUR CHILD IS DIAGNOSED WITH ATTENTION DEFICIT DISORDER

"Jimmy seems like he has been on the go ever since he could walk. As soon as he hit one-year-old, we started chasing him. It was like he had a non-stop motor going all the time. He had trouble going to sleep, slowing down, getting along with other kids, and now his teacher says he has to see someone because he is so hard to control in his new kindergarten class. One-on-one we have had some success, but as soon as he is in a group setting like school all the trouble begins. He does not listen like the other kids, he bullies the smaller ones, and he just gets silly. Does he need medication?"

Attention Deficit Disorder ranks among the most frequently diagnosed behavior disorders. ADD affects about 8 percent of school aged children in the United States.

The syndrome is characterized by more than expected degrees of:

INATTENTION

Trouble focusing on activity
Trouble sustaining attention
Seeming not to listen
Trouble following instructions
Easily distracted

Easily bored
Trouble organizing
Making careless errors
Not finishing homework
Losing things
Not doing homework
Not following instructions
Having to have things repeated

IMPULSIVITY

Inability to wait her turn
Blurting out answers in class
Interrupting
Bossiness
Acting like the class clown
Having little control of his actions and not being able to put thought between feelings and actions
Having hair-trigger tempers
Bullying

HYPERACTIVITY

Trouble sitting still
Fidgeting
Rarely slowing down, always on the go
Talking too much
Rarely finding quiet time

It's true that many of these characteristics are, to some degree, common to all children. This in no way lessens the validity of the disorder. A child's capacity to focus, sit still, follow commands, control activity, show patience, and manage feelings develops at different rates. There is no such thing as a perfectly normal timeline and because of this, it's important not to jump to conclusions.

But by kindergarten these areas of development should be growing, and by the first and second grade, they should be well along. If not, then chances are she is in a great deal of discomfort and might be suffering from ADD.

Three Types of Add

There are three types of Attention Deficit Disorder:
Attention Deficit Hyperactivity Disorder (ADHD) where the hyperactive/impulsive characteristics predominate.
Attention Deficit Disorder (ADD) where inattention predominates and there are fewer behavioral problems characteristic of children with ADHD.
Combined Type where there are both inattentive and hyperactive/impulsive characteristics.

Children with ADHD often get into more trouble than their peers. These are the children who precipitate those evening calls home. The teacher will complain that the child seems not to listen and clowns around, or that she becomes distracted easily and will daydream. Parents often report that these children are "spacy," don't have any interests, and have behavioral problems at home as well as in school. Parents will often tell me that, now that they remember, their newly diagnosed child was into things even as a toddler with a motor that never turned off. They'll tell me about excessive dangerous climbing, running off, tripping, clumsiness, and say that the child has been a handful for years. These children often have trouble learning as well.

ADD can lead to other problems

As bad, if not worse, than the syndrome itself are some of the secondary problems that untreated children with ADD can develop, including:

Poor self-esteem or depression
Feelings of exclusion and alienation from peers
Anxiety
Learning disabilities
Conduct disorder
Oppositional defiant disorder
Tics or Tourette's syndrome

If untreated, these children also have a higher rate of:
Teenage substance abuse
Antisocial behaviors
Car accidents
Ending up less accomplished in nearly all areas

What causes it?

We don't know what causes AD(H)D. Some think that it might be inherited. Others have linked AD(H)D with low levels of lead in a child's blood, and still others to cigarette smoking and alcohol use by the pregnant mother. Some have hypothesized that early, stress-related parenting problems interfering with bonding might be a significant cause. And, of course, theories about sugar and even food additives abound, but are so far unproven. We do not know the cause of AD(H)D, but luckily that doesn't make the problem any harder to treat.

Diagnosis

The diagnosis of AD(H)D is best made by a child psychiatrist. There is no particular psychological or blood test to diagnose the disorder. The most effective way to know if a child has AD(H) D is by gathering a history of the child's functioning from parents, teachers, and others who interact with her, and from the child herself. Thus, a lengthy history gathering is necessary. Care has to be taken to rule out other disorders that can look similar, especially anxiety disorders and depression with agitation, as well as post traumatic stress disorder. Sometimes children react to situational changes with AD(H)D-like behavior, but this is usually passing and not long-term like AD(H)D. Many parents are quick to point out that many AD(H)D behaviors seem to disappear in one-on-one settings or when a child is in front of a television or computer. Such comments do not rule out AD(H)D since these children are most symptomatic in larger and somewhat less organized settings like school or camp. Lastly, the psychiatrist looks to see if the behaviors are present in more than one setting, as they usually are. If the behavior is only present in one setting, then the doctor should figure out if that particular setting is triggering anxiety.

Treatment

Once the diagnosis is made, a multimodal or combination approach is usually necessary including some form of therapy such as:
Behavior therapy
Individual talk therapy
Educational help
Family therapy
Parent education
Skills training
Medication

Remember that therapy for the secondary effects of AD(H)D listed above is every bit as important as treating the syndrome itself. These co-morbid (which simply means existing simultaneously) disorders need to be treated as well.

Medication treatment of ad(h)d with stimulant drugs

Medication is one of the core treatments for AD(H)D and has a history in child psychiatry going back over fifty years. Although stimulant medications are by far the most effective and widely used drugs, currently the treatment of AD(H)D also includes other classes of psychotropic medications. These are far less effective but might be necessary when stimulants don't work or cannot be tolerated. These medications will be considered further in other chapters but are also mentioned below. They include antidepressants, blood pressure medication, antipsychotics, mood stabilizers, and anticonvulsants.

AD(H)D medications have received a lot of publicity over the years, mostly because of the millions of children who have received them. Reports have ranged from raves about their effectiveness to diatribes against their safety that instill the fear of death in parents. In fact, these medications are the most widely used in child psychiatry and have been the most studied, so they are some of the safest medications out there. The stimulants are not only effective agents to treat AD(H)D, but also work quickly with very few troubling side effects.

How effective is the medication?

Stimulants help about 75 percent of children who take them for AD(H)D. That's a pretty good response rate. The other 25 percent might benefit from other medications and interventions. Although the stimulants best affect the behavioral components of AD(H)D syndromes, many other aspects of the child's functioning improve as well.

How does it work?

These medications are thought to work by altering transmitters—dopamine and norepinepherine— in the central nervous system, making them more available or more effective. The exact mechanism is not known. Essentially, though, the stimulants increase alertness and arousal, giving a child with ADD increased attentional capacity, better focus and memory, increased organization, better concentration, and less restlessness and overactivity. She will be less impulsive and thus easier to deal with in school and at home. Listening to authority figures will improve, homework and learning will be easier, and there will be less fighting with peers and family members.

What are the side effects?

Common, usually mild, and often transient side effects are decreased appetite, minimal weight loss, reversible very small decreases in height, headache, abdominal pain, insomnia, mild irritability/anxiety, and weepiness. Your child might get one or two of these and they will be slight and manageable. The younger the child, the worse and more common the side effects may appear, and thus smaller doses are usually given.

It was once feared that height problems might persist over time but that has been disproven. There was also concern that these medications could cause irreversible tics. While it's true that they can cause tics in rare cases, they resolve after reducing or stopping the medication. In some families where tics are more common, greater care is taken in prescribing stimulants. Other concerns include the medication affecting blood cell count, which happens only rarely, and very rarely psychotic symptoms such as hallucinations and delusions occur in children with predispositions to psychotic disorders. I have seen only one case of this in decades of prescribing for an uncountable amount of children. Great care has to be taken in prescribing for children with psychotic tendencies.

There has been some recent publicity about the possibility of sudden cardiac death associated with stimulant use. One study concluded that there is a quite rare chance of such an occurrence. The study has since come under question. Well-known medical organizations dispute the findings and consider the chance of sudden death in children on stimulants as rare an event as in the general population of children. While it is true that these drugs cause a negligible heightening of the pulse rate and blood pressure in some children, they are very safe, especially in children with no pre-existing heart disease. Therefore, it is essential that the psychiatrist get a history of any cardiac symptoms to rule out any possible undiagnosed cardiac conditions. Some people have recommended the routine use of ECGs (electrocardiograms) to detect silent cardiac diseases including certain rhythm disturbances and heart muscle abnormalities, but this recommendation does not seem warranted. What is warranted is a good history of the child, asking about symptoms of cardiac disease such as chest pain, shortness of breath, fainting, seizures, palpitations and the like, as well as a thorough physical examination by the pediatrician. In the absence of a family history of cardiac disease, especially sudden death in the family, or symptoms of such disease in the child (such as a condition called cardiomyopathy, long QT syndrome seen on an ECG and other diseases), there is little evidence for the utility of routine ECG's or consultation with a cardiologist for a child about to start stimulant medication. If during treatment cardiac symptoms appear—again, chest pain, shortness of breath, etc.—then you should be referred to a cardiologist.

WHAT ARE THE MEDICATIONS AND HOW ARE THEY USED?

Stimulant medications abound. The two major classes of stimulant are methylphenidate (i.e. Ritalin) and its derivatives, and

Amphetamine (i.e. Adderall) and its derivatives. The following are the most common stimulants listed by trade name followed by chemical name and peak concentration times and duration of action:

TABLE 1
METHYLPHENIDATE COMPOUNDS

BRAND NAME	**GENERIC NAME**	**DURATION OF ACTION (IN HOURS)**
RITALIN	METHYLPHENIDATE	PEAK 2 LASTS 3-4
RITALIN-SR	METHYLPHENIDATE (SUSTAINED RELEASE)	PEAK 4.7 LASTS 7
RITALIN LA	METHYLPHENIDATE (EXTENDED RELEASE)	PEAK 2 AND 6 LASTS 8-12
CONCERTA	METHYLPHENIDATE LONG ACTING	PEAK 1 LASTS 8-12
DAYTRANA PATCHES	METHYLPHENIDATE	PEAK 7 LASTS 10
FOCALIN	DEXMETHYLPHENIDATE	PEAK 2 LASTS 3-4
FOCALIN XR	DEXMETHYLPHENIDATE	PEAK 2 AND 6 LASTS 10
METADATE	METHYLPHENIDATE	PEAK 2.5 LASTS 8
METADATE CD	METHYLPHENIDATE BEADS IMMEDIATE AND LONG ACTING	PEAK 1.5 AND 4 LASTS 8-12
METHYLIN	METHYLPHENIDATE ORAL AND CHEWABLE	PEAK 1-2 LASTS 4
METHYLINE ER	METHYLPHENIDATE TABLETS	PEAK 4 LASTS 8

TABLE 2
AMPHETAMINES

BRAND NAME	GENERIC NAME	DURATION OF ACTION (IN HOURS)
DEXEDRINE	DEXTROAMPHETAMINE	PEAK 1-2 LASTS 4-6
DEXEDRINE SPANSULES	DEXTROAMPHETAMINE	PEAK 1-4 LASTS 6-10
DEXTROSTAT	DEXTROAMPHETAMINE	PEAK 2 LASTS 10
DESOXYN	METHAMPHETAMINE	PEAK 3 LASTS 10
ADDERALL	2 AMPHETAMINE SALTS	PEAK 1-3 LASTS 5
ADDERALL XR	2 AMPHETAMIONE SALTS EXTENDED REALEASE	PEAK 1-4 LASTS 9
VYVANSE	2 AMPHETAMINE SALTS LINKED TO LYSINE	PEAK 3.5 LASTS TO 12

Which ones are approved for children?

All the stimulants are approved for children six years old and over. Adderall, Dexedrine, and Dextrostat are also approved for children as young as three years old. There has been some concern in the media about use of stimulants in children under six years old. While it is true that these younger children might have more side effects at lower doses than older children, their use in this age group has been growing as the medication's ability to help some young children has become clear. In general, it has been my habit to withhold medication from these younger children unless the benefits will clearly outweigh the risks. In a case, for instance, where the child is disruptive to the point of not being able to attend school, or impossible to discipline, and so to withhold treatment would be harmful and possibly even dangerous. It almost seems like a miracle to watch these medications rapidly relieve or ameliorate a child's symptoms. The effect of stimulants in adolescents, while quite good, is a bit less dramatic than in school age children (six to twelve years old) but that is no reason to withhold these medications from teenagers. On the contrary, their use in adolescents continues to be a cornerstone of treatment.

How many children take these medications?

About 3 percent of school-aged children currently receive stimulant medication.

How are the stimulants prescribed?

Each psychiatrist develops his own style of prescribing within the overall safe parameters of the profession. I try to be as flexible as possible. After I explain to the child and his parents about AD(H)D and how medication can help, I try to ascertain the family attitudes as well as that of the child, attempting to decrease any resistance or fear. I point out that the child is usually just as smart as his peers although he might not think so due to chronic failure. I explain what we are trying to accomplish by describing the target symptoms we want to alleviate. I point out that the medications are remarkably safe, but I do say that there is a chance of mild and transient side effects, which I describe, but not in so much detail to arouse anxiety and even suggest their presence. I explain that I will be available with any questions and will be following the course of treatment on a regular basis.

Before beginning treatment with a stimulant, it is wise for the psychiatrist to be sure thc following have been done:

1. A full history has been obtained with special focus on any history or family history of tic disorders, seizures, and any particular heart disease symptoms in the child and family.

2. Measurements of height and weight.

3. Blood pressure and resting pulse.

4. Baseline blood tests including, at a minimum, a complete blood count and liver function tests.

5. An EKG only if the aforementioned cardiac issues are present.

6. A full pediatric physical examination and, in best of all possible worlds, agreement with the pediatrician about the use of medication.

I usually start with a short acting form of methylphenidate (see below for list of short and long acting stimulants) such as Ritalin. I want this given on a weekend day at first so parents are around to observe any untoward reactions and make initial observations about any positive effects. The short-acting compounds work fast and are eliminated from the body quickly so any side effects will abate rapidly. After this initial weekend dose I suggest a starting dose for school days. The usual prescription is for two doses—one in the morning before breakfast and another before lunch. These doses start low and are increased until the optimal dosage is found. The increases occur no more frequently than once a week. Sometimes there is a need for a third dose. The longer acting drugs make any school administration unnecessary which, for some children, helps avoid the embarrassment of taking medication at school. I usually recommend no medication be taken on weekends or on vacations unless the clinical condition warrants it. If methylphenidate doesn't work, I usually switch to an amphetamine compound. On the whole, the goal is to switch to long-acting compounds whenever possible. For those children in whom a long-acting dose wears off in the late afternoon, it is suggested that a short-acting dose be used so homework can be done, but not so much or so late that insomnia ensues.

How long will my child have to take the medication?

In general, if there has been a good response, I suggest that each year we consider stopping medication over the summer, if possible, and then restart it if school dysfunction arises again. Other psychiatrists suggest starting medication again at the end of the summer so as to avoid school failure in the fall and then withdraw it after a month or so to see if it is needed anymore and thus not risk trouble at the beginning of the school year.

It is important that the child is followed up regularly with medication evaluation sessions. At first these are done monthly at least as the child's dosage becomes individualized. After several months the visits can become less frequent but never less than quarterly.

TABLE 3
SHORT ACTING STIMULANTS

BRAND NAME	AVAILABLE DOSAGES (MGS)
RITALIN	5, 10, 20
DEXEDRINE	5, 10, 15
FOCALIN	2.5, 5, 10
ADDERALL	5, 7.5, 10, 12.5, 15, 20, 30
METHYLIN	5MGS/5CC 500 CC BOTTLE

TABLE 4
INTERMEDIATE ACTING STIMULANTS

BRAND NAME	AVAILABLE DOSAGES (MGS)
RITALIN SR	20
METADATE ER	10, 20 , 30, 40, 50, 60
DESOXYN	5

TABLE 5
LONG ACTING STIMULANTS

BRAND NAME	AVAILABLE DOSAGES (MGS)
RITALIN LA	10, 20, 30, 40
CONCERTA	18, 27, 36, 54
DAYTRANA	10, 15, 20, 30
FOCALIN XR	5, 10, 15, 20, 30
METADATE CD	10, 20, 30, 40, 50, 60
ADDERALL XR	5, 10, 15, 20, 25, 30
METHYLIN ER	10, 20
DEXEDRINE SPANSULES	5, 10, 15
VYVANSE	20, 30, 40, 50, 60, 70
DEXTROSTAT	5, 10

When Stimulants Fail

Not all children respond well to stimulant medications. Luckily, there are other drugs available, although they are usually not as effective as the stimulants. If both methylphenidate and amphetamine compounds fail, the next drug of choice is Straterra (Atomoxetine), an antidepressant thought to increase available levels of norepinepherine, as well as possibly dopamine, in the brain. It is usually given once a day and does not require controlled substance prescriptions like the stimulants, thus refills can be given. Rapidly absorbed, it peaks in the blood in about two hours. Abdominal pain, nausea, headache, and decreased appetite are the main side effects. Because it is an antidepressant, there is a warning on the box about increased suicidal ideation. This will be discussed below in the chapter on antidepressants, but suffice it to say that this is a disputed finding and one which I have never witnessed in any child as a result of antidepressant use.

In addition to Straterra, other antidepressants of the tricyclic class have been used to treat ADD and also Wellbutrin. In addition, there has been success using antihypertensive drugs such as Clonidine and Tenex (often in combination with a stimulant) which will also be considered elsewhere in this book. Lastly, for severe ADD which does not respond to stimulants, many psychiatrists are having success using antipsychotic medication and even mood stabilizers. These latter medications will be discussed in separate chapters

CHAPTER FOUR

ANTIPSYCHOTIC MEDICATION

"My husband and I are on the verge of panic. Our son was seeing a psychiatrist for what we thought was ADHD. He gave him Ritalin and then Adderall but they didn't help. Rob kept on getting suspended. Today we had a follow up appointment and the doctor suggested giving him Risperdal. We got home and looked on the computer and it said that Risperdal is an antipsychotic. Our son has problems but he's not psychotic! Now we don't know what to do and need a second opinion."

"But Dr. Paul you said Marie had bad tics and was not seriously disturbed and now you suggest an antipsychotic medication. Are you suggesting she's schizophrenic?"

"Mark is just depressed, not crazy. Why are you putting him on Abilify? I read that's an antipsychotic for schizophrenics. Are you saying my son is schizophrenic?"

Of all the drug classifications, antipsychotics sound the scariest to parents. They assume that by prescribing them, the doctor is saying their child is psychotic. It's essential to understand that this class of drug—in spite of its name—has many uses and has helped countless children with different disorders. Unlike stimulants, which essentially treat one mental disorder—ADD --antipsychotics are used in the treatment of not only psychoses (disorders which include the loss of touch with reality), as their name implies, but for many behavioral problems in children and teens.

These drugs are called antipsychotics because upon their introduction into mainstream psychiatry they were used primarily for the psychoses. But as time has passed, this has been greatly overshadowed by their widespread use treating myriad other conditions. Unfortunately, the name has stuck and thus the immediate anxiety parents, and teenagers, experience when they are suggested. Many parents simply won't give it to their children just because of the label. Until someone comes up with a more suitable name, parents need to be educated and reassured.

THE DISORDERS

Antipsychotics are, to many, miracle drugs because of how effectively they can correct or greatly ameliorate myriad disorders, from schizophrenia to tics to the more difficult behavior disorders. They can also be used as adjunct therapy for depression when an antidepressant alone isn't enough.

Schizophrenia

As mentioned, though their usefulness is widespread, antipsychotics were first used to treat the severely mentally ill. *Schizophrenia*, the most well-known of the psychotic disorders and among the most serious that a psychiatrist encounters, is characterized by:

- Hallucinations (hearing voices or seeing things)
- Delusions (often bizarre and odd beliefs like feeling people are out to harm them or thinking that they are famous)

- Disorganized speech and behavior
- Hard to understand outbursts of feelings.
- A flattening of feeling
- Odd relatedness in social interaction (tendency to make communication difficult or bizarre laughing at serious moments)
- Difficulty working
- Suspiciousness
- Neglect of appearance
- Withdrawal and decreased motivation, amongst other things

Before the development of these drugs this devastating disorder would often necessitate long-term institutionalization. When these drugs were introduced in the 1950's, the population of people in hospitals greatly diminished, as it became possible to live in the community free of some of the disabling symptoms of this disease. These drugs continue to be the cornerstone of treating seriously disturbed adults and teenagers and have revolutionized modern psychiatry. Schizophrenia is rare before adolescence with the typical onset in late adolescence or early adulthood.

Psychotic Disorders other than schizophrenia

More common than full-blown schizophrenia in children and some adolescents is a condition in which there are psychotic symptoms such as auditory hallucinations and odd thinking which does not quite meet all the formal criteria for schizophrenia. It is not as highly structured a syndrome. It might go away or develop later into a full blown psychotic diagnosis. This is often called *Psychosis, nos* (not otherwise specified). Another non-schizophrenic psychotic disorder found in adolescents more than children (but mostly in young adults) is called *Brief Psychotic Disorder*. It is relatively short lasting (hours to days) characterized by hallucinations, delusions, thinking that is disorganized, confusion, memory problems, sometimes strange language, disorientation, a high degree of emotionality, and sometimes unusual dress and behavior. There is often a clear trigger—an event—that starts such an episode (death of a loved one, assault), though not always. Both of the above conditions respond to antipsychotic medication.

Conduct Disorder and Oppositional Defiant Disorder

Today Antipsychotics are most commonly used to treat serious behavior disorders in children such as Conduct Disorder and Oppositional Defiant Disorder.

Conduct Disorder (CD) is characterized by:

- Persistent breaking of rules
- Aggression toward other people/animals
- Fighting, bullying, cruelty, intimidation
- Destruction of property
- Fire setting
- Lying
- Stealing
- Other law/rule breaking
- Running away
- Truancy
- Breaking curfew

Typically these behaviors begin just before or after the onset of puberty. Conduct Disorder is serious and often a forerunner of the adult Sociopathic/Antisocial Personality.

Oppositional Defiant Disorder (ODD) is a characterized by:

- Negativism
- Rebellion
- Arguing
- Defiance
- Anger episodes
- Revenge
- Resentment
- Spite
- Annoying others
- Blaming others
- Irritability
- An overall passive aggressive stance ("I will show my anger by not doing…")

In addition to adolescent schizophrenia and behavior disorders in both children and teenagers, antipsychotics are used frequently in the treatment of:

Stimulant-resistant Attention Deficit Hyperactivity Disorder
(See Chapter Three)

Not all young people with ADHD respond to the stimulants or antidepressants used in treating that disorder. In these cases, antipsychotics are used quite successfully. In fact, the use of antipsychotics for this non-psychotic disorder is becoming quite prevalent. This should not scare you. It does not mean that your child is seriously impaired. She is just in that group of non-responders to the routine ADHD medications and thankfully the antipsychotics can help.

Tics (including Tourette's syndrome)

A tic is a repetitive body movement or vocal utterance which is repetitive, quick, sudden, non-rhythmic, and uncontrollable, although it can be suppressed for a short time. Tics can occur in any part of the body—eye blinking, rapid movements of the head, neck, limbs, torso, face, and shoulders. There are also vocal tics such as throat clearing and other sounds or even words. Most of the time tics are mild and transient although sometimes they are more severe and long lasting. A diagnosis of Tourette's Syndrome is given when both motor and vocal tics have occurred in the same child. Antipsychotic medication is a first line treatment for serious tic disorders.

Childhood bipolar disorder

This disorder is characterized by periods of depression and mania (elevated mood, grandiosity, irritability, flight of ideas, rapid speech, and motor hyperactivity) in adults and recently has become a more popular diagnosis in young people. There is controversy about whether in fact true bipolar disorder exists in children. But antipsychotic medication is helpful in major disorders of behavior in which some characteristics of mania exist, especially the symptom of irritability when it is severe and long lasting. Unlike adult bipolar disorder, there is less or no cycling of depression and mania. There is a lot of anger and trouble-making, rapid mood changes, impulsivity, anxiety, sleep problems, and problematic interpersonal behavior. Many people find it difficult to differentiate these behaviors from AD(H)D. Others feel that these children, with such a wide variety of symptoms, simply represent a problem with mood regulation and the latest psychiatry diagnostic manual has proposed a new category of Temper Dysregulation with Dysphonia (depression) syndrome which can describe these children. But regardless, the antipsychotic medications can help in controlling some of these behaviorally difficult children.

Certain behavioral aspects of Autism (Pervasive Developmental Disorder). Autism is a complex syndrome characterized by:

- Impaired social relatedness
- Lack of social reciprocity
- Decreased peer relationships
- Sharing deficits
- Delayed or lack of language
- Odd/repetitive speech
- Poor conversational skills
- Rigidity
- An obsessive need for sameness
- Rituals
- Motor mannerisms
- Preoccupations with parts of objects or narrow interests

Antipsychotic medication has only proven helpful in a narrow range of these problems including irritability, tantrums, some of the motor issues, the occasional high anxiety of these children (sometimes to the point of psychosis), and repetitive behaviors. Unfortunately, there is little pharmacological help for the core of Autism, which is impaired communication and decreased relatedness.

Agitation

This symptom can be found in many mental disorders such as psychosis, depression, anxiety states, and developmental disorders. Antipsychotics help with agitation independent of the source disorder.

Self Injurious Behaviors

Self-burning, cutting, scratching, hair pulling, wound-picking, injecting oneself, and other injurious behaviors are most common in adolescents who have another diagnosis as well. These are all disorders of impulse control and can occur across a host of psychiatric diagnoses such as Borderline Personality Disorder, mental retardation, and severe mixed depressive/anxiety states. Antipsychotic medications help in all these conditions.

Behavioral problems associated with Post Traumatic Stress Disorder (PTSD)

Many children who have been abused, exposed to domestic violence, sexually violated or neglected, will often present with syndromes which have a high level of severe misbehavior, anxiety, agitation and aggression, all of which commonly respond to antipsychotic medication.

Severe Eating Disorders

Bulimia and anorexia will often respond to antipsychotics when other therapies have failed.

Other severe mood and anxiety disorders

Antipsychotics are often the second line of defense for illnesses that don't respond well to antidepressants or antianxiety agents.

TRENDS IN USE OF ANTIPSYCHOTIC MEDICATION

Antipsychotics were introduced into psychiatry in the 1950's and came to be called first generation antipsychotics. They did wonders to relieve the symptoms of psychotic people but had many unpleasant side effects. The most typical side effects were the mimicking of certain neurological disorders—specifically Parkinson's Disease, amongst others—thus these early drugs were also called *neuroleptic drugs* (inducing neurological symptoms) or typical antipsychotic medication.

In the 1990's newer drugs called second generation antipsychotic drugs were introduced which caused fewer of the typical neurological side effects—thus they are also called *atypical antipsychotic drugs*. These drugs not only had fewer side effects than the original drugs, but were also considered to be somewhat more effective in treating the negative symptoms of schizophrenia rather than just the positive symptoms like hallucinations and delusions. These negative symptoms include such phenomena as decreased spontaneity, facial inexpression, monotone speech, and overall difficulty in living actively engaged in the tasks and enjoyment of life. These newer atypicals, as they are called, have drawn great attention as they are used more and more in psychiatry—including in children and adolescents—than are the first generation. These newer atypicals account for about 90 percent of the antipsychotic prescriptions made to young people today.

The rate of prescribing these drugs has grown astronomically as they have become a mainstay for child and teenage psychiatrists. Studies have shown a growth rate anywhere from 80 to 500 percent depending on the study. Not only have these drugs been used more but have been shown to be effective for childhood disorders that were very difficult to treat before especially in the area of psychotic syndromes and aggressive disorders. The greatest increase in use has been in the age group of seven to eighteen years old but there have been increases in usage even in the preschool category.

HOW OFTEN ARE THEY PRESCRIBED?

Since these drugs are mostly prescribed off label and can also have serious side effects (see below), they have come under scrutiny and criticism. There have been myriad headlines, internet stories, and even what appear to be politically motivated congressional inquiries into the increased use of these drugs. While it is appropriate to keep well abreast of any risks of medication, it is important to understand that once the media gets a hold of information it is often exaggerated, and much of the so-called information on the internet is questionable at best, fallacious at worst. Still, these valuable drugs continue to be prescribed in increased numbers, helping hundreds of thousands of children cope with disabling mental disorders. Due to their potential side effects it is essential that a skilled child psychiatrist be the prescriber and that certain safeguards be built into the treatment (see below).

HOW DO THESE DRUGS WORK?

The antipsychotic medications, both typical and atypical, are thought to work in the central nervous systems as blockers to neurotransmitters. Specifically, the first generation drugs act mostly by blocking the receptors that receive the transmitter called dopamine. The second generation antipsychotics block the effects of dopamine and serotonin. Some of the other antipsychotics, like the newer Abilify, are thought to act by only partially blocking dopamine and serotonin receptors and mimicking dopamine and serotonin action but in a much lower and modified way.

WHAT ARE THE NAMES OF THE DIFFERENT TYPES OF ANTIPSYCHOTIC MEDICATION?

What follows is a listing of the different antipsychotic medications, their brand and generic names, the ages for which they have been approved, and the available dosage forms. Not every available antipsychotic will be listed as many are used only rarely and over the years newer products have replaced the original typical ones.

First Generation Typical Antipsychotic Medications

There are many Typical Antipsychotics. The most well-known and most often used are listed here. Still, as mentioned above, these are used only rarely as compared to the Atypicals.

TABLE 6
TYPICAL ANTIPSYCHOTICS

BRAND NAME	GENERIC NAME	APPROVED FOR AGES	AVAILABLE DOSAGES (MGS)
HALDOL	HALOPERIDAL	AS YOUNG AS AGE 3 YEARS OLD	TABLETS .5, 1, 2, 5, 10, 20
THORAZINE	CHLORPROMAZINE	AS YOUNG AS ONE YEAR OLD	TABLETS 10, 25, 50, 100 , SYRUP, SUPPOSITORIES
MELLARIL	THIORIDAZINE	AS YOUNG AS 2 YEARS OLD	TABLETS 10, 15, 25, 50, 100, 200
STELAZINE	TRIFLUOPERAZINE	18 YEARS OLD	TABLETS 1, 2, 5, 10
NAVANE	THIOTHIZENE	18 YEARS OLD	TABLETS 1, 2, 5, 10, 20
MOBAN	MOLINDONE	18 YEARS OLD	TABLETS 5, 10, 25, 50

Like the Atypicals, these drugs are all similarly effective in treating psychotic and behavioral symptoms. Their major side effects, however, have decreased their popularity.

Second Generation Atypical Antipsychotic Medications

These medications are becoming extremely popular and are used for a host of conditions mentioned above. They are extremely effective and don't have many of the disabling side effects of the Typical Antipsychotics, making them the preferred therapeutic agents for a host of conditions. The following are the most well-known and most often used.

TABLE 7
ATYPICAL ANTIPSYCHOTICS

BRAND NAME	GENERIC NAME	APPROVED AGES	AVAILABLE DOSAGES (MGS)
RISPERDAL	RISPERIDONE	AS YOUNG AS AGE 10 YEARS OLD	.25, .5, 1, 2, 3, 4
ZYPREXA	OLANZAPINE	AS YOUNG AS AGE 13 YEARS OLD	2.5, 5. 7.5, 10, 15, 20
SEROQUEL	QUIETAPINE	AS YOUNG AS 10 YEARS OLD	25, 50, 100, 200, 300, 500
CLOZARIL	CLOZAPINE	18 YEARS OLD	25, 100
ABILIFY	ARIPIPRAZOLE	AS YOUNG AS 10 YEARS OLD	2, 5, 10, 15, 20, 30
INVEGA	PALIPERIDONE	18 YEARS OLD	1.5, 3, 5, 9
GEODON	ZIPRASIDONE	WILL SOON BE APPROVED FOR 10 YEARS OLD	20, 40, 60, 80

SIDE EFFECTS OF THE TYPICALS

- **Sedation** Fatigue or sense of sleepiness
- **Parkinsonism** This side effect mimics the symptoms of Parkinson's Disease with rigidity of muscles, a shuffling gait, a hand tremor when at rest that looks like one is rolling pills, a fixed facial expression, lack of arm movements while walking, a cog wheeling feeling when moving the limbs, slowness of movement, decreased spontaneity emotionally and physically, and a decreased control of movement under volitional control.
- **Dyskinesia** These are bodily movements which the individual cannot control. It happens most often around the muscles of the face (mouth, jaws, tongue) and arms which are either regular, slow, and done in some rhythmic fashion or irregular. Some patients develop ataxia (lack of coordination) or apraxia (inability to carry out learned movements). This disorder is sometimes called *tardive dyskinesia* as it often occurs only slowly after years of treatment.
- **Dystonias** This is an earlier occurring disorder and includes contractions of muscle groups (spasms) sometimes even resulting in abnormal postures. Included here is torticollis (twisted neck), eyes rolled up under the lids, rapid eye blinking, mouth and tongue spasms, and spasms of the larynx and esophagus.
- **Akasthisia** An unpleasant sensation of motor restlessness, anxiety, inability to sit still, tension, and sometimes insomnia.
- **Seizures**

ATYPICALS ALSO HAVE THEIR SIDE EFFECTS

The Atypicals were developed and became the preferred antipsychotic medications because they have so many fewer of these neurological side effects. Although there are some treatments for the side effects of Typicals—stopping the typical or adding medications (medications such as such as benadryl, artane or cogentin, Inderal and drugs of the anti-anxiety class such as Klonopin (clonazepam) for agitation—the Atypicals have soared in popularity as they usually avoid the effects in the first place. While the Typicals have their specific, well-known side effects which initiated the search for antipsychotics with less trouble and gave birth to the widespread use of the Atypicals, other side effects have arisen from these drugs which warrant our attention and need to be watched for.

Specifically the Atypicals are associated with the possible development of:

• **Metabolic Syndrome** This is conglomeration of conditions which heighten one's risk of developing heart disease and diabetes. Specifically these conditions are:

- Rise in blood triglycerides
- Decrease of good cholesterol
- Increased weight
- Increased blood pressure
- Increased fasting blood sugar

So while there is less sedation and neurological side effects, the fear of these metabolic abnormalities has caused great concern.

• **Elevated Prolactin Levels** can be caused by all antipsychotic medications, but now that children and teenagers are taking so much more of the Atypicals there is a heightened concern and association between the Atypicals and prolactin levels. Prolactin is a hormone that is a natural substance in the body and aids in breast preparation during pregnancy and for milk production after birth. There are certain medical disorders that can cause Prolactin to increase at other times. The use of antipsychotic medication can cause it as well. In adults, hyperprolactinemia can lead to abnormal menstrual cycles, infertility, lactation, and erectile dysfunction. In studies, children with antipsychotic-induced high prolactin levels haven't experienced any definitive long lasting negative effects but the levels are followed with blood tests. My female patients have occasionally experienced embarrassing incidents of lactation as well as menstrual abnormalities, and the males some mild breast enlargement. In these instances I have switched to medications with fewer of these effects. But in general, high prolactin levels have not yet been proven to have long-lasting deleterious side effects in young people. I do follow the blood levels of prolactin though, to be on the safe side, and to monitor for excessively high levels. Nearly all children who get elevated prolactin levels develop normally, and if a problem occurs it is easily corrected.

- **Elongated QTC Interval On The EKG** is an abnormality which has drawn attention recently. The EKG essentially is an electrical tracing of the hearts muscular contractions. The main electrical complex is composed of the Q, R, S, and T waves. Some medications elongate the time interval between the Q wave and the T wave (the QTC interval) which means that the preparation of the heart for its next beat is prolonged. This has been associated with the development of rhythm disturbances one of which, torsade de pointes, can be fatal. In fact, a prolonged QTC often comes from other conditions, sometimes a genetic predisposition and from drugs including antipsychotic medication—typicals and atypicals. It has become of interest lately because of the increased use of Atypicals. Interestingly, studies have not shown definitive evidence linking antipsychotics to an elongated QTC and sudden death but safety dictates that the psychiatrist take measures of prevention. That is why, before starting antipsychotic medication,

I require an EKG with a QTC reading. If it is prolonged to a dangerous level I usually will not prescribe the drug. If it is somewhat elevated or if it is normal I will prescribe but track the QTC regularly, at least semi-yearly, throughout treatment. If it becomes elongated, it usually does so slowly and there is time to stop the medication. In all my years of prescribing antipsychotics to hundreds of young people I have never seen a clinical problem and only saw two cases of a slight increase in the QTC. Thus, I consider these medications safe from a QTC viewpoint.

- The Atypical antipsychotic medications are thought to exert their effects somewhat through antagonizing the effects of serotonin and acetylcholine and thus are associated to a small degree with causing agitation and anxiety, as well as drowsiness, headache, dry mouth, low blood pressure upon standing, insomnia, constipation, and increased heart rate.

POSSIBLE SIDE EFFECTS OF BOTH TYPICAL AND ATYPICAL ANTIPSYCHOTICS

The most serious of the possible side effects from both typical and atypical antipsychotics is **Neuroleptic Malignant Syndrome,** a rare but dangerous condition. The symptoms include a high fever and muscle rigidity, confusion, excessive sweating, abnormal blood pressure, irritability, agitation, and even delirium and coma. If your child has any combination of these symptoms get her to the emergency room.

Other occasional side effects of all antipsychotic medications include:

- Constipation
- Dry mouth

- Decreased urination
- Behavioral problems
- Irritability
- Depression
- Apathy
- Rapid heart rate
- Fainting associated with low blood pressure upon getting up from bed or from sitting
- Severe reactions to sun exposure
- Severe blood abnormalities like agranulocytosis, especially with Clozapine from the Atypical group of drugs
- Eye abnormalities
- Liver abnormalities

WITHDRAWAL

If one stops taking any antipsychotic drug there is always the chance of a withdrawal syndrome including dizziness, nausea, vomiting, sweating, insomnia, anxiety, shaking, agitation, and some have even reported hallucinations. Unless there is need for emergency cessation, for instance, in the cases of acute muscle spasms (dystonia) any psychotropic medication must be withdrawn slowly.

MEDICAL EXAMINATIONS ESSENTIAL FOR CHILDREN AND TEENS TAKING TYPICAL AND ATYPICAL ANTIPSYCHOTICS

Because of the relatively high number of possible side effects from antipsychotics, both typical and atypical, it's important that your child's doctor do the following:

1. Height Measurement
2. Weight measurement

3. Blood tests including a complete blood count, blood chemistries including liver function tests, fasting blood sugar, levels of lipids including total cholesterol, good cholesterol (HDL), bad cholesterol (LDL), serum triglycerides, and kidney tests (blood urea nitrogen levels [BUN] and creatinine levels).
4. EKG with QTC reading.
5. Blood pressure and pulse.
6. A physical exam to include an examination for any abnormal movements.
7. These tests should be repeated at six month intervals.

HOW MANY CHILDREN TAKE THESE MEDICATIONS?

It is unknown how many children take these medications since most are given off label prescriptions, making it difficult to get an exact figure. We do know that the numbers have increased since their usefulness in treating so many disorders has become widely understood. One estimate I read put the number at about 7/1000 children and teenagers which would translate to 500,000–1,000,000 children and teenagers.

HOW EFFECTIVE ARE THESE DRUGS?

Despite the rapidly growing use of the Atypicals and the long history of the Typicals in psychiatry, there are few reliable studies attesting to the effectiveness of this class of medication, although we know beyond a doubt through clinical practice that they are extremely effective. There have been many studies, but flaws in the studies have been pointed out. Many patients do not adhere to the study protocols or are lost to follow up. In young people, almost all of the drugs are used off label and studies about effectiveness are scant. It has been my personal experience that these drugs are quite effective in treating most of the aforementioned mental disorders. Unlike stimulant studies though, a precise percentage of positive responders in each diagnostic category is not available at this time. What can be said is that for the most part the successful use of these drugs outpaces use of a placebo nearly all the time. These medications are most effective in psychotic disorders, stimulant resistant ADHD, other disruptive behavior disorders—especially those with aggression and irritability, and as adjuncts in depressive disorders, anxiety disorders, and agitation—and in mania. They are less effective in Conduct and Oppositional Defiant Disorder, eating disorders, and self injurious disorders, but could be of some help so they should be tried if your doctor prescribes them.

HOW ARE THESE DRUGS USED?

Nearly all studies of these drugs have been with adult populations and thus dosage requirements for children and teens have not been clearly defined. In general, I start with the lowest possible dose and very slowly titrate upward until achieving a therapeutic effect, a goal which has been spelled out prior to treatment. Of course, the incidence of side effects will often limit the use of a particular drug. Thus the well-known slogan: "start low and go slow."

I tend to stay away from the typical antipsychotics because of the side effect profile above. The one exception I make is with tic disorders because they respond so well to Haldol. Some doctors find, however, that Risperdal works just as well. I will also use a typical in cases of severe agitation where sedation is needed for the patient to be safe. In general, though, I usually start with an Atypical medication. I use Risperdal the most, as it has been prescribed to young people the most. Although it has not been proven to be more effective than the other Atypicals, I favor it over Zyprexa and Seroquel because there are hints that these drugs might cause more metabolic effects. This has not been fully proven but has been the impression of many. Other child psychiatrists prefer other antipsychotics and here, as in medicine as a whole, a combination of knowledge and personal style/preference dictates which drugs are used. I use Abilify mostly as an adjunct for depression treatment when an antidepressant medication needs augmentation or when there is a definite diagnosis of bipolarity. It has also been my experience that Abilify, in some cases, might cause a bit of agitation/anxiety and insomnia more than others. When this is the case I make sure it is given in the morning to avoid insomnia and I discontinue it if the agitation/anxiety is severe. I have very rarely used the Atypical Clozaril which is considered by many to be the most effective antipsychotic, because of the risk of agranulocytosis, a rare but sometimes fatal blood cell side effect.

Again, the amount of Antipsychotic medication to be given when treating the aforementioned mental disorders has not been itemized. One cannot say with accuracy which disorder gets how much antipsychotic. In general, psychotic conditions usually necessitate a higher dose than do the other disorders and it takes a bit longer to ameliorate the symptoms. In general, I see positive effects within the first week of treatment of children and teens with behavioral disorders. For schizophrenic children (with delusions and hallucinations) it usually takes weeks. For psychotic children other than those with schizophrenia, response rates are more rapid as well.

WHEN ANTIPSYCHOTICS FAIL

An antipsychotic might fail to help your child. Occasionally, more patience is needed as the psychiatrist raises the dose, although with most of these drugs raising the dose above set limits only causes more side effects without helping much. Sometimes another drug has to be tried. It is rare that I will ever use two antipsychotic drugs simultaneously except when changing over for days or weeks. But the use of two of these drugs simultaneously on a consistent basis usually does not increase effectiveness. It has been my experience that if a correct diagnosis has been made then an antipsychotic will help: often, though not necessarily, the first one. We do not know why one medication might work better in a particular child than another. That is a mystery yet to be solved.

CHAPTER FIVE

ANTIDEPRESSANTS

"At first our eight-year-old Ivan's teachers thought he had ADHD. He would stare off, seemed consumed with daydreams, and never paid attention to his work. But one day he told his gym teacher that he was just too sad to participate in basketball and that he was always sad and lonely. Now I feel that my wife and I misread his crying in his room as a reaction to poor grades but maybe he's just been depressed all these years. After all, he never seems to really enjoy anything for more than a few minutes, drops new hobbies, and rarely gets excited."

"Joanne seemed sad and withdrawn when she heard about her friend Sally's leukemia. We figured, "Who wouldn't be?" After ten days she seemed worse. She stayed in her room listening to Gregorian chants, started reading the Bible, and didn't eat or even come out. Last night she said she felt guilty that she didn't get sick herself. She said we would be better off without her around and wrote a poem about the joy of death."

For many years the psychiatric establishment didn't believe that children could experience depression. We saw depressed children every day, but because many of the theories that informed our work implied that children had not reached a developmental stage capable of getting depressed, we could not call them depressed.

This backward thinking stopped much research and development of treatments for childhood depression. We now know this was shortsighted. As the stories above, and hundreds of thousands like them, attest, children and teenagers of all ages experience depression. Still, tragically, the great majority of these youngsters do not get proper evaluation or treatment due to limited availability of care and lack of compliance with treatment. This leads to high levels of family, educational, and social problems, as well as substance abuse and other psychiatric problems, and even suicide—one of the leading causes of death for adolescents in this country.

Young People Do Get Depressed

Like adults, children and teenagers have a wide variety of feelings. In fact, young people often seem to have more frequent changes of mood than adults, varying from day to day, hour to hour, even minute to minute. Sadness, joy, excitement, frustration, irritation, exuberance, sulkiness, anger, and the like are all normal and add to the colorful picture that defines us as people. Our inborn temperaments affect our overall capacity to feel, express ourselves, respond to others, regulate ourselves, and in general they give each child a biological range of moods which forms a backdrop to how a child grows and interacts. Family influences also affect how children express feelings.

In the normal course of life there are many events which cause sadness: disappointments, loss of family or friends, moving, failures and successes, and social setbacks, to mention a few. This is normal. Sadness is usually self limited to hours, days, or a week or two, and goes away as a child moves on and continues to participate in and enjoy the many challenges of being alive. Sadness, like so many feelings, is part of life and should not be interfered with by parents. In fact, a bit of sadness and withdrawal allows each of us to regroup, grow, and get ready to face other challenges.

But a depressed child or teenager is different from one who is simply sad. Six per cent of young people are depressed at any one time and depression is a high risk marker for suicide. Thus, childhood depression is a great health challenge for our country. Depressed children and teenagers often appear as if their personalities have changed. While sadness is normal, it is also experienced as more superficial than the more painful and deeper feelings of depression. While a sad child might experience a bit of frustration and disappointment, a depressed one is often angry, irritable, cranky, whiny, and prone to rage at times, even violence. Sleep and appetite patterns change, weight is lost, menstruation and normal bowel function are affected, personal appearance deteriorates, and serious fatigue could ensue as well.

Sad children and teens don't lose self esteem, but depressed ones do, often feeling like they are bad, losers, worthless, unlikable, and inferior in a host of ways. Frequent crying without a cause is not uncommon. Depressed young people often feel sick and have a host of pains—headaches, stomach aches, and muscle stiffness. They will often feel hopeless, a particularly worrisome sign that is associated with suicide. School functioning decreases as concentration, attention, and attendance drop off. These kids will usually isolate from friends and families. Communication is lessened and often irritation in short spurts is all that a parent sees. Formerly fun activities give little pleasure and are sometimes replaced by risky pursuits and behavior. Energy is low and fatigue is high. These depressed youngsters often look like they move in slow motion, heads down, slumped shoulders, with a sad and pained expression. They appear to be apathetic. Sometimes a depressed child talks of running away or becomes angry at authority.

Suicidal thoughts and even, tragically, successful attempts are not uncommon.

About four million children and adolescents suffer from some form of depression at any time in the United States. Fortunately, this is a treatable condition if properly diagnosed.

The Statistics of Suicide

Of course, suicide is always a worry when there is talk about depression. While suicide is quite uncommon for younger children, we do see an increase starting at about nine years old. By thirteen to fourteen years old, the rate of suicide increases and, as mentioned above, is the third highest cause of death for 10–24 year olds. The rate of suicide under ten years old is about .8/100,000 children, it doubles in the 10–14 year old group, but then increases to about 8/100,000 by 15–19 years old. Suicide attempts are often reported as accidents and are not reflected in the statistics—like the depressed teenager who crashes the car into a tree. About two thousand suicides in youngsters occur in the United States each year. There are about one hundred thousand world-wide. While depression is the main risk factor associated with youth suicide, other conditions also raise the risk:

- Behavior disorders
- Physical/sexual abuse
- Severe anxiety
- Eating disorders
- Suicide in the family
- Substance abuse
- Being bullied
- Family disruption

Triggers

There are many triggers for suicide including being rejected socially or in a love relationship, school failure or expulsion, being caught by the police doing an antisocial act, feeling humiliated, being intoxicated, and experiencing family stress. But hopelessness, often found in depressed youngsters, is one of the most indicative signs of a possible suicide attempt.

Warning Signs

Potentially suicidal young people frequently show warning signs. What follows is a list of some of the thoughts, feelings, and actions that could indicate that a young person is contemplating suicide. They range from internal, unexpressed thoughts, like wanting to die, to overt actions, like writing a note or collecting drugs or weapons.

- Thoughts of death
- Wanting to die
- Prior suicide attempts/gestures
- Feeling that the world would be better off if they were dead
- Feeling useless and hopeless
- Giving verbal hints about not being able to take it anymore
- Writing about death
- Getting absorbed in music, video sites, or activities stressing death or suicide
- Talking of the afterlife
- Dressing in black
- Becoming absorbed in morbid subjects
- Having an inappropriate burst of enthusiasm or cheerfulness after being depressed (this sometimes indicates that a person has decided to commit suicide)

- Cleaning house and putting his/her things in order
- Writing a suicide note
- Buying books or researching modes of suicide
- Idealizing celebrities who have committed suicide or died in other ways
- Engaging in drunken driving
- Accumulating weapons

What to Do About Suicide Concerns

The *most important* thing you can do when you are concerned your child is thinking about suicide is to explore the situation openly. If your child states that he has suicidal ideas or intentions or plans then an immediate mental health evaluation is necessary. But things are often not that clear. First ask yourself, "Is my child or teenager depressed?" If after a week or two, a sad mood does not budge or gets worse and signs of depression are present, be concerned. Talk to your child openly about how he or she is feeling. Include direct questions about suicide. Many parents mistakenly feel that by asking about suicide they will put it in a child's mind. This does not happen. It is important to know what your child is thinking and direct questioning is the best way to find out. You can ask directly about suicidal ideas, rehearsals, preparations, and the like. This can also be done by asking something like: "Sometimes when we feel like this, thoughts of dying or wanting to take your own life can pop up. Has that ever happened to you?" Further probing can include other questions like:

- Do you think about death?
- Do you feel like you want to disappear?
- Do you feel hopeless?
- Do you think about the afterlife?

It is also essential that you look for possible signs of preparation: a note or other writing, a weapon, or hoarded medication. If, after open, kind, and compassionate questioning of your sad child, without lecturing or criticizing, you see no progress in the depression, and have little or no handle on understanding the situation, and see any signs of possible suicidal intent, then a mental health assessment is needed. No time should be wasted in getting professional attention.

Sometimes we must take more urgent/emergency measures if such a young person becomes defensive, angry, aloof, withholding, and even outright violent at your attempts at helping. At that point outside help is mandatory. After removing any dangerous items such as pills, weapons, or other items that might be used self-destructively, you must talk directly to your child about your concerns. Not talking openly about suicide sometimes makes the situation more dangerous. The professional evaluation can be done in a private office of your doctor or mental health professional or in the emergency room of a hospital. The teenager or child might resist this strongly with shouting, attempts to intimidate, running away, and even physical violence. If that happens, you must call in outside help such as 911 to ensure your child's welfare. Remember that his/her defensive behavior is an attempt to ward off exposure, further humiliation, or embarrassment, but you are trying to ward off the tragedy of suicide. Your child deserves the highest level of your concern. Getting help will be looked back upon with gratitude some day.

TREATING DEPRESSION WITH MEDICATION

The Black Box Warning

The use of antidepressants has come under great scrutiny in the past six years due to warnings that were issued by the Federal

Drug Administration. A 2003 report and another started in 2005 found that antidepressants possibly lead to increased suicidal thinking and even suicidal behavior in young people. In 2007 the FDA decided to mandate the following black box warning, so called because it is printed in a black box on the medication:

WARNINGS: SUICIDALITY AND ANTIDEPRESSANT DRUGS

Antidepressants increased the risk compared to placebo of suicidal thinking and behavior (suicidality) in children, adolescents, and young adults in short-term studies of major depressive disorder (MDD) and other psychiatric disorders. Anyone considering the use of [Drug Name] or any other antidepressant in a child, adolescent, or young adult must balance this risk with the clinical need. Short-term studies did not show an increase in the risk of suicidality with antidepressants compared to placebo in adults beyond age 24; there was a reduction in risk with antidepressants compared to placebo in adults aged 65 and older. Depression and certain other psychiatric disorders are themselves associated with increases in the risk of suicide. Patients of all ages who are started on antidepressant therapy should be monitored appropriately and observed closely for clinical worsening, suicidality, or unusual changes in behavior. Families and caregivers should be advised of the need for close observation and communication with the prescriber.

This was put on all antidepressants although the studies had only been done for some SSRI depressants (see below). This warning, and the accompanying publicity, scared parents and led to a marked decrease (up to 50 percent) of antidepressant prescription for young people, Prozac excluded (this was the only antidepressant approved for children). This happened in spite of the fact that it was stated that no one should stop their antidepressant and that there had been no suicides in the group studied.

After the black box warnings came out, much was written about the fact that it was almost impossible to know if the depression itself caused the suicidal trends and not the medication. The study showed that possibly 4 percent of young people developed these suicidal trends (no actual suicide) compared to 2 percent amongst those who were not treated. Many psychiatrists, including myself, appeared on national news shows emphasizing that if, in fact, this was a risk, it was so rare that most of us had never even seen it, and that proper monitoring by the prescribing physician would in all probability be enough to ward off any tragedy. Despite this, the new prescribing of antidepressants dropped markedly. Tragically, the suicide rate increased in teenagers. No scientific correlation was made, but it seems that this was related to less use of the antidepressants which could have treated the depression and prevented the suicide.

As it stands now, the anxiety about antidepressants has decreased. To my knowledge, there have been no further studies leading to alarm. Prescribing has increased again and it appears that most prescribers are more vigilant about monitoring for this side effect.

If prescribed correctly, under the guidance of an experienced professional, I do not think there is a particularly significant increased risk of suicide. Further studies about particular drugs with proper control groups will clarify the situation. I would not advise any parent to withhold antidepressants based on what we know so far. But be cautious and make sure your child is being monitored for every possible side effect.

Medication Alone Is Never Wise

For the treatment of depression to be successful, it must include some form of the many psychotherapies available, be it individual, family, and/or group. It can be plain old psychodynamic talk therapy or cognitive-behavioral therapy, social support, self-help groups, supportive counseling, life counseling, or social skills aid. Many studies going back years have shown that treatment for depression combining therapy with medication leads to the best outcome. In today's world, with limited numbers of child/adolescent psychiatrists and mental health professionals in general, and with much of the prescribing being done by non-psychiatric physicians, many children are just being given a pill. I implore parents to seek help from a health care provider who uses or recommends verbal therapy to accompany the use of medication.

How Antidepressants Work

Like antipsychotic medications (see Chapter Four) these drugs have come to be used for more than depression. Antidepressants are thought to work by altering neurotransmitters in the central nervous system. Until the 1950's doctors used opiates and stimulants to treat depression. Around that time doctors started researching an anti-tuberculosis drug called Isoniazid and a related compound called iproniazid and found that they reversed sedation caused by certain drugs and also stimulated depressed people. The modern era of antidepressants began. It was not clear how these original compounds worked, but it was felt that they inhibited the breakdown of certain natural body enzymes which in turn broke down certain chemicals in the body which were involved with maintaining a good mood. These breakdown enzymes were called monoamine oxidases, and thus the first antidepressants were called monoamine oxidase inhibitors or MAOI inhibitors. These are still in existence but have been overshadowed by later discoveries of medications with less troublesome side effects. Next were the tricyclic antidepressants, so named because there are three rings in their chemical structures. Imipramine was the first one and was derived from work with antihistamines. Imipramine was thought to act by increasing the availability of the neurotransmitter norepinepherine in the central nervous system. In the next two decades the neurotransmitter serotonin also became a focus for scientists. Antidepressants thought to selectively increase the availability of serotonin in the central nervous system became and remain the most popular drugs in the antidepressant class: the selective serotonin reuptake inhibitors or SSRI's.

Presently about one million antidepressant prescriptions are written yearly in the United States for young people. This number has quadrupled in the last several years. In general, the antidepressants are used off label in children except for the following:

- **Prozac** approved for depression in children eight years old and over for depression;
- **Anafranil** approved for children ten years old and older but for Obsessive Compulsive Disorder only;
- **Lexapro** approved for twelve to seventeen year olds for depression;
- **Luxox** approved for eight year olds for Obsessive Compulsive Disorder only;
- **Sinequan** approved for twelve year olds for depression;
- **Tofranil** approved for six years old and over for bedwetting only;
- **Zoloft** approved for six year olds for Obsessive Compulsive Disorder only.

Thus, seven of the twenty-nine known antidepressants are approved for children and only three for depression. Despite that, these drugs are used widely and safely for many children across the country.

A Closer Look at Types of Antidepressants

MAOI Inhibitors

The MAOI inhibitors include: Marplan, Nardil, and Parnate and newer ones among which is called Aurorix. *These drugs are rarely if ever given to young people. I have never used them with children or teenagers.* They were found to be effective in depression and ADHD. These compounds essentially increase a host of neurotransmitters including norepinepherine, serotonin, dopamine, and phenylethylamine. They increase the effects which mimic the sympathetic nervous system and thus cause an increased heart rate and blood pressure. Due to this effect, when a person eats food high in tyramine the drug stops its metabolism and this can lead to what is called a hypertensive crisis with severely elevated blood pressure. This is known as the cheese reaction because of the high levels of tyramine found in certain cheeses. A diet low in tyramine and tyramine-like compounds must be strictly followed when taking MAOI inhibitors and thus one has to avoid aged cheese, cured or aged meats, fava bean products, yeast extract, sauerkraut, soy sauce, bean products, tap beer, certain wines, sausage, bologna, pepperoni, and salami, all of which have high levels of tyramine. Other foods with tyramine have to be eaten in moderation only: avocados, caffeine, chocolate in large amounts, large amounts of peanuts, raspberries, and spinach. Considering these restrictions and side effects, I feel these drugs are better left off the list of desired drugs for children, except in extreme circumstances when no other drug(s) has worked.

Tricyclic Antidepressants

These compounds were the most popular antidepressants until about twenty years ago when the SSRI's were introduced (see below). These compounds, like the other antidepressants, are thought to mediate the effects of the neurotransmiters, including norepinepherine, dopamine, serotonin, and acetylcholine. Tricyclics increase these transmitters at the cellular level in the central nervous system.

The most widely used tricyclics are (see chart below):

- **Anafranil- particularly effective in obsessive compulsive disorder**
- **Aventyl**
- **Elavil**
- **Ludiomil**
- **Norpramin**
- **Sinequan**
- **Surmontil**
- **Tofranil—used widely for wetting syndromes**
- **Tofranil PM**
- **Vivactil**

Tricyclic medications have been found to be useful in the following conditions:

- Depression in teenagers and children
- ADHD
- Enuresis (Bedwetting, defined as voiding of urine into bed or clothes, during the night or day or both, twice a week for three months or causing significant distress, in a child of at least five years)
- Aggression

- Anxiety Disorders (see chapter on anti-anxiety drugs)—including school phobia, panic disorder, obsessive compulsive disorder, separation anxiety, and hair pulling (trichotillomania)
- Certain behaviors often found in Autism such as self-destructive behaviors, rituals, and other stereotyped behaviors

Although the tricyclic antidepressants were extremely popular and are still used to some extent, there were side effects that proved troublesome to many patients.

The most common side effects of Tricyclic antidepressants are:

- Increased heart rate and blood pressure
- Some changes in the EKG; linked to this were reports of sudden death in six children taking Norpramin and a few with tofranil, although it was never proven that these deaths were related to EKG changes such as slowed conduction. Before starting your child on this drug, the doctor should get a baseline EKG and follow up every six months.
- Blurred vision
- Dry mouth
- Trouble urinating
- Constipation
- Sexual functioning problems
- Drowsiness
- Drops in blood pressure when getting up from sitting or from bed (orthostatic hypotension) due to effects on blood pressure
- Weight gain
- Minor liver dysfunction including jaundice
- Very rarely: disorientation, memory loss, delirium, shaking, sweating, abdominal pain, and even psychosis.

People who stop these drugs abruptly might also suffer from a flu-like withdrawal syndrome. This is quite rare and includes mostly nausea, vomiting, and headache as well as some irritation. These drugs should be tapered over at least a two week period if stopping.

More serious, and one of the main reasons these drugs have become overshadowed by the newer SSRI group of antidepressants, is that overdose with Tricyclics can be very dangerous, even fatal. Accidental childhood poisoning with these drugs is high. In overdose these drugs are toxic to the conduction of electricity in the heart. An overdose of these drugs is a medical emergency requiring immediate hospital care in most cases.

Before starting Tricyclics, it is especially important to have a full physical exam including an EKG so that pre-existing heart issues are discovered which will lead to closer observation if necessary.

In general, I tend to avoid these drugs as first choice for depression due to the side effects. Although I have never been convinced that they have been proven to be associated with sudden cardiac death, the necessity of following EKG's and the slight chance of causing cardiac arrhythmias places it as a second choice in my practice. I do, however, use it regularly for enuresis because of its effectiveness.

Selective Serotonin Reuptake Inhibitors (SSRI's)

The SSRI's are now the most commonly used anti-depressants in the United States. Their supposed mechanism of action is to increase quantities of the neurotransmitter serotonin in the nerve synapses in the brain by inhibiting the reuptake of this chemical by neurons which secreted it (the presynaptic neurons). These medications help not only with depression but are also used to reduce anxiety and inhibit aggression. They are so popular because

they have a better side effect profile than the tricyclics and are safer in the event of an overdose. Not as fatiguing, they also produce less dry mouth, constipation, dizziness, and fewer urinary problems. Some people experience uncomfortable gastrointestinal side effects including nausea and diarrhea and something called behavioral activation—disinhibition that presents as an increase in disruptiveness, anxiety, and a feeling of agitation. Some patients also describe an internal driven-motor feeling as a side effect.
The most common SSRI's are (see table below):
Celexa
Lexapro
Luvox—Especially effective in obsessive compulsive disorder
Paxil
Prozac
Zoloft—Especially effective in post-traumatic-stress disorder and other anxiety states

Like the tricyclics, these drugs are used for more than depression. They are also used for:

- Anxiety syndromes
- Post traumatic stress disorder
- Obsessive compulsive disorder
- Some of the behavioral problems and irritability found in autism

If one discontinues an SSRI there might be what is called an *SSRI discontinuation syndrome* mainly consisting of dizziness, bad dreams, nausea, and vomiting.

Another danger of using SSRI's is the *very rare* possibility of developing what is known as the *Serotonin Syndrome.* This a syndrome characterized by some of the following: agitation, sweating, shivering, shaking, diarrhea, fever, lack of coordination, confusion and agitation, rapid heart rate, high blood pressure, and hallucinations. It is caused by a rapid elevation of serotonin and can be caused by ingesting one drug like an SSRI or a combination of drugs (more common), an overdose of a drug, or even the use of illicit drugs. One must stop using the drug(s) causing it and be managed medically either at home, if this is mild, or in a hospital by treating the symptoms. This syndrome is potentially fatal if serious and untreated. Most people get better soon after stopping the use of a particular drug. The following drugs are considered suspect in producing this side effect:

- Antidepressants
- Opioid drugs
- Central nervous stimulants
- Psychedelic drugs
- Certain herbs like St. John's Wort

Norepinepherine-Serotonin Reuptake Inhibitors

This type of antidepressant works through increasing both serotonin and norepinepherine in the central nervous system. Some feel that these medications might be a bit more effective than SSRI's but that is far from proven in studies. Because of their similarities to SSRI's they share many of the same side effects (including serotonin syndrome and a discontinuation syndrome), but because of their mode of actions on norepinepherine, hypertension, especially, becomes more of a concern.

The most common SNRI's are:
Cymbalta
Effexor, effexor xr
Pristiq
Savella

These drugs are also used to treat:

- Depression
- Anxiety disorders
- Pain syndromes like fibromyalgia
- ADHD
- Obsessive compulsive disorder

Other Antidepressants

WELLBUTRIN—A second line antidepressant that is often used as an augmenter when other antidepressants need a boost. It is also somewhat effective in stimulant resistant ADHD.

TRAZADONE—This is not a particularly effective SSRI-like antidepressant but does cause a high degree of sedation. That is why it is used as a sleep agent more than anything. It is particularly used by adult drug addicts with insomnia because it avoids using potentially addictive sleep agents in this population.

SERZONE—Like Trazadone, this is an SSRI-like antidepressant which is rarely used due to worries about severe liver problems.

REMERON—Another rarely used antidepressant which has found most of its use based on its lack of sexual side effects. It is rather weak as an antidepressant.

How Effective are Antidepressants?

There is controversy about the degree of effectiveness of antidepressants compared to placebo when treating depression. While we know that they work up to about 60 percent of the time for people with major depression, we are not sure how well placebos do. Some say the difference is great while others say only small. One of the reasons for this is that many studies are short term, include groups of patients with varying diagnoses, have a high drop-out rate, poor follow ups, and use scales which differ at different parts of the studies. My impression is that antidepressants work well for young people who have been properly diagnosed with major depression as well as those with a bona-fide anxiety disorder (including post-traumatic-stress disorder, obsessive-compulsive disorder, and other anxious states), enuresis (bedwetting), and for some depressive/anxious symptoms found in autistic children. Since in clinical practice it is difficult to withhold medication from people who are suffering, I cannot say whether placebo, or the passing of time, compares with active treatment. But I do know from taking of histories from people who have suffered without proper treatment for months and years, these medications, when introduced, significantly ameliorate long time pain.

How are Antidepressants Prescribed?

As mentioned above, nearly all of the antidepressants are prescribed off label as are most psychotropic drugs in general. Below I list the antidepressants by category and list the available dosages manufactured. In general, if I choose to use an antidepressant in a young person I start at half the adult dose. This is in contradiction to what is known—that children usually metabolize drugs faster and thus the half life of compounds is shorter. Despite that I feel that there is more to be known about children and these drugs so the safest route is to start even lower than might be advised. Constant and frequent monitoring will allow the prescriber to measure how fast to increase dose as the side effect/clinical effect ratio is observed.

The general rules for antidepressant prescribing for depression is as follows: In practice I usually start depression medication by using an SSRI. If that does not work well, I can switch to another SSRI. If that does not work, I can either switch to a TCA which I have done often or try to augment the initial drug(s). Augmentation means while keeping the child on an original non-effective or partially effective antidepressant I add an augmentation agent such as: wellbutrin (considered as a second line antidepressant), Lithium (see chapter on mood stabilizers), thyroid hormone, buspar (see chapter on anti-anxiety medications), an atypical antipsychotic—especially abilify (see chapter on antipsychotic medication), stimulants (see chapter on stimulants), or benzodiapines (see chapter on anti-anxiety medications). This type of polypharmacy has become more common over time and is now considered regular practice.

The Common Antidepressants

(I do not list the MAOI's, as they are rarely, if ever, used in young people; approved dosages are only listed for those FDA approved for children).

TABLE 8
TRICYCLIC ANTIDEPRESSANTS

BRAND NAME	GENERIC NAME	AVAILABLE DOSAGES (MGS)
TOFRANIL	IMIPRAMINE	10, 25, 50
TOFRANIL PM	IMIPRAMINE	75, 100, 125, 150
ANAFRANIL	CLOMIPRAMINE	25, 50, 75
ELAVIL	AMITRIPTYLINE	10, 25, 50, 75, 100, 150
PAMELOR	NORTRIPTYLINE	10, 25, 50, 75
NORPRAMINE	DESIPRAMINE	25, 50, 75, 100, 150
SINEQUAN	DOXAPINE	10, 25, 50, 75, 100, 150
SURMONTIL	TRIMIPRAMINE	25, 50 100
VIVACTYL	PROTRIPTYLINE	5, 10

TABLE 9
SSRI ANTIDEPRESSANTS

BRAND NAME	GENERIC NAME	AVAILABLE DOSAGES (MGS)
CELEXA	CITALOPRAM	10, 20, 40
LEXAPRO	ESCITALOPRAM	5, 10, 20 PLUS LIQUID PREP.
LUVOX	FLUVOXAMINE	25, 50, 100
PAXIL	PAROXETINE	10, 20, 30, 40
PROZAC	FLUOXETINE	10, 20, 40 PLUS 90 WEEKLY
ZOLOFT	SERTRALINE	25, 50, 100

TABLE 10
SNRI ANTIDEPRESSANTS

BRAND NAME	GERNERIC NAME	AVAILABLE DOSAGES (MGS)
CYMBALTA	DULOXETINE	20, 30, 60
EFFEXOR	VENLAFAXINE	25, 37.5, 50, 75, 100
EFFEXOR XR	VENLAFAXINE EXTENDED RELEASE	37.5, 75, 150
PRISTIQ	DESVENLAFAXINE	50, 100
SAVELLA	MILNACIPRAN	12.5, 25, 50, 100

TABLE 11
OTHER ANTIDEPRESSANTS

BRAND NAME	GENERIC NAME	AVAILABLE DOSAGES (MGS)
WELLBUTRIN	BUPROPRION	75, 100 MGS
WELLBUTRIN XL EXTENDED RELEASE	BUPROPRION	150, 300
WELLBUTRIN SR SUSTAINED RELEASE	BUPROPRION	100, 150, 200
DESYREL	TRAZADONE	50, 100, 150, 300
SERZONE	NEFAZADONE	50, 100, 150, 200, 250
REMERON	MIRTAZAPINE	15, 30, 45

CHAPTER SIX

MOOD STABILIZERS FOR BIPOLAR DISORDER AND OTHER CONDITIONS

"The first psychiatrist we saw about Bobby's behavior said he had a behavior disorder, while the second said it was ADHD. Now we are told he has Bipolar Disorder. But he doesn't seem like the descriptions I read of people with that problem. We are pretty confused especially since each doctor wants to try a different medication. What should we do?"

"My son Randy has been having behavior problems for years. We took him to the University clinic and he received his fourth diagnosis called TDD. My wife and I don't know what's going on and we can't find out what those three letters mean."

"Our family has had many with Bipolar Disorder. Our daughter Margo just had a major bout with depression but the hospital mentioned she might really have Bipolar Disorder because of her bad temper. They said because of that her treatment would be different than if she only had regular depression."

Bipolar Disorder (BD) is a disorder of mood. Called "bipolar" because the mood varies between the two poles of mania and depression, the condition affects about .5 to 4 percent of the adult population, depending on the diagnostic criteria used. That figure has been pretty steady over time. What has changed has been the number of children, pre-adolescents, and early adolescents diagnosed with BD recently. These numbers have skyrocketed, causing debate about whether, in fact, all these children suffer from true BD. While we know that mid and later-adolescents often suffer from forms of BD similar to those in adults, children younger than this can present with a wide variety of more vague, generalized, and diffuse symptoms. We are not sure of the exact number of correctly diagnosed children but do know for sure that the numbers have increased from 400 percent to 4000 percent depending on the criteria used. Thus, the number of children receiving medication for BD has also skyrocketed, despite the fact that diagnosis of childhood BD is still an evolving phenomenon.

What Does Bipolar Disorder Look Like in Adults?

Originally BD was called Manic Depressive Illness since it was characterized by episodes of mania and depression, often presenting as discrete episodes of illness with mostly normal intervals in between. The present APA manual of diagnosis defines BD as a mental disorder in which an individual suffers from at least one episode of mania or what is called a mixed episode (mania and depression together) and also usually has had separate episodes of depression as well. Depression has been defined in chapter five, so here we will concentrate on the definition of mania and its less serious counterpart known as hypomania.

A **manic episode** lasts at least a week and is essentially a disturbance during which the person has an unusually elevated, expansive, and/or irritable mood which is not usual for the person.

In addition, the person might have at least three or four of the following:

- Too rapid speech
- Less of a need for sleep
- Inflated ideas about himself, called "grandiosity"
- The tendency to be more talkative than usual in a pressured manner and with rapidity
- A feeling of racing thoughts
- Difficulty being followed by others
- Excessive energy
- Distractability
- Physical agitation
- Involvement in potentially destructive activities like sexual promiscuity or spending too much
- An apparent increase in goal-directed activities at work, socially, sexually, or at home (excessive cleaning that keeps him up all night)
- Psychosis, with hallucinations and delusions which are an extension of the mood disturbance—like expansively thinking s/he is a world renowned figure from history, a famous athlete, a genius, a great inventor etc.

Manic episodes cause marked trouble for the person and can often result in breakdown in work, family, and social functioning. Hospitalization is sometimes necessary.

A hypomanic episode is very similar to a manic episode except it never involves hallucinations and delusions, must only last four days and not a week to be diagnosed, and does not cause as great a disturbance in functioning, although others usually notice a difference in behavior.

BD is usually characterized as Bipolar 1, 2, and Cylcothymia. Bipolar 1 Disorder involves at least an episode of mania and often periods of depression as well. The episodes tend to be distinct but sometimes include mixed episodes of mania and depression. Bipolar 2 disorder is a form of BD with periods of depression and at least one episode of hypomania. Cyclothymia is a mood disorder with periods of abnormal moods that are a bit less than hypomania and less serious depression as well. In addition to Bipolar types 1 and 2, mixed episodes, and Cyclothymia, many clinicians see varied forms of disordered moods that don't fall into neat categorization. These are called Atypical bipolar disorders or soft bipolar disorder. In addition, we sometimes see hypomanic or manic episodes which might have been caused by an antidepressant, but this is quite rare. Some researchers say that it is simply a depressed person previously unknown to have bipolarity coincidentally developing the next stage (mania or hypomania) when he was being treated with an antidepressant drug.

What Does Bipolar Disorder Look Like in Children and Young Teens?

The adult presentation of BD as it is historically known begins to appear in mid to late adolescence. In younger children, classical BD is extremely rare. In dealing with literally thousands of children I have come across only a handful of cases of classical BD. The upsurge in diagnoses has occurred in younger children because these children present with behavior disorders associated with mood changes that are hard to classify using the present diagnostic parameters. But including them in the BD category might not be the solution.
For example:

- In childhood one rarely encounters the above mood episodes (mania/hypomania and depression) as separate distinct entities. In other words, it is difficult to identify discreet episodes of elevated or irritable mood episodes, intervening normal periods, and then discreet episodes of depression. In children who have mood variability with characteristics of bipolar episodes there is usually no cycling as there is with adults and the course is much more variable. In fact, it is rare to see full blown mania in young children, keeping in mind that there are normal times when children seem to feel great or even overly exuberant as a regularly occurring reaction to an external event or personal achievement.

- Since in adulthood irritability frequently presents as part of a manic episode, the psychiatric community decided to put children with excessive irritability alternating with other mood variations in the category of BD. But this seems more like convenience for the diagnostician than truth. If all these children were in fact presenting with forms of BD then they would eventually develop true BD, which they do not.
- Many children classified as Childhood BD really suffer from AD(H)D, a disruptive behavior disorder other than ADHD, Post Traumatic Stress Disorder with behavioral disorder, or plain severe anxiety. Even youngsters with hypersexuality (typical of mania) often are sexually abused children acting out.
- It appears to me that behavior disordered children who don't quite fit the AD(H)D, Oppositional Defiant Disorder or Conduct Disorder entities have been deposited in the BD category for lack of a better fit. And since some of the medications used for BD help with excessive behaviors, the diagnosis is made.

In summary, truly Bipolar children are a rarity in clinical psychiatry although, on occasion, one does see such a child. More likely, your child who has a severe behavioral disorder, great variation in mood, resistance to medications for ADHD, or anxiety is suffering from a mixed disorder which defies strict diagnosis at this time. The good news is that there is treatment for these children.

TDD

A new syndrome has been identified that might be included in the next addition of the psychiatric diagnostic manual: It is called Temper Dysregulation Disorder with Dysphoria or TDD. Newly described, but known to many of us for years, this classification has been suggested to replace the diagnoses of many so-called bipolar children. These children can be described as:

- Having frequent tantrums in response to stress
- Acting with rage and aggression out of proportion to whatever the cause
- Having behavior that makes them appear younger than they really are
- Experiencing these episodes at least several time a week
- Feeling a lot of irritability, anger, and sadness (dysphoria) in between tantrums
- Having tantrums that appear in more than one setting (home and school) and starting before ten years old and no earlier than six years old

These symptoms generally have to last a year to officially be called TDD.

TDD makes itself known quite frequently. These children also share other characteristics:

- They do not have mania.
- They share a similarity to children with Oppositional Defiant Disorder.

- They rarely develop BD but are more likely to become depressed as they get older if not treated. I have often seen depressed adults who describe their behaviors as children that sound like TDD.

Medications for BD, TDD, and Accompanying Conditions

Children younger than mid-adolescence rarely present with classically described Bipolar Disorder. Therefore, the available treatments are those for adults, used off label for children. The medical establishment calls the group of medications Mood Stabilizers. Other than Lithium, the most well known of the group, most of the mood stabilizers were used originally by neurologists to treat epilepsy and are called anti-epileptic medication. These medications are often used in conjunction with Antipsychotic medications for children with BD and TDD. Although formal studies are somewhat lacking, it does seem that these drugs help. For the sake of discussion we will address the BD child as one who either presents as having classic BD (rare) or TDD.

How Do We Treat BD and TDD?

The treatment of BD in children is similar to that of Adult BD. First, we treat whatever the episode is being experienced—acute phase treatment—and when things get better we focus on preventing future episodes—maintenance phase treatment. Most of the medications for both phases are the same. One must also keep in mind that BD children often have comorbid (additional) diagnoses which might need treatment as well.

Acute Phase Treatment

The acute phase of treatment of BD means medicating a child who is either manic, depressed but with a bipolar history (bipolar depression), or one who has TDD.

The initial acute phase treatment for mania without psychotic features (hallucinations and delusions), or TDD starts with monotherapy-treatment with one drug. The one drug is either a **mood stabilizer** such as Lithium, Depakote, or Tegretol, or less commonly Gabapentin, Trileptal, or Topamax; or an antipsychotic drug (see Chapter 4) such as Risperdal, Seroquel or Zyprexa, or less commonly Abilify or Geodon. If the child only partially responds then an augmenting agent is often tried in conjunction with the first medication. Usually this consists of adding an antipsychotic to a mood stabilizer or conversely a mood stabilizer to an antipsychotic. Alternatively, if the child does not respond to monotherapy the psychiatrist sometimes skips the augmentation phase and just switches to another of the original choices of monotherapy listed above. Again, there is then the opportunity to add an augmenter here as well. If the child still fails to respond then differing combinations of mood stabilizers and antipsychotics are often tried. On the whole most children do respond to one or more of the more common first line drugs (Lithium, Tegretol, Depakote or Risperdal, Seroquel or Zyprexa).

For BD children with psychotic features it now common to start right off with a combination of a mood stabilizer (Lithium, Depakote, or Tegretol) and a more common antipsychotic drug. If this fails at first one can switch the combination of mood stabilizers and antipsychotic medications; then one can add another antipsychotic medication or add another mood stabilizer. Finally, if all combinations of the common mood stabilizers and antipsychotics are exhausted, one can use the less effective of the mood stabilizers in conjunction with different antipsychotic medications.

Bipolar Depression is major depression in a person who has had either mania or hypomania in the past. The most effective acute phase treatments in adults (there are few studies in children) are Lithium and Lamictal—two mood stabilizers that have antidepressant effects in Bipolar depressives. The use of the usual antidepressants (see Chapter 5) is frowned upon to a degree—not only because they are only partly effective, but also because the SSRI group in particular might actually cause problems by increasing agitation and causing unwanted destabilization. Some psychiatrists also use Wellbutrin as this is considered to be a weaker antidepressant but one that does not cause bipolar cycling as much as traditional antidepressants—although it has never been proven that increased cycling is ever caused by antidepressants at all.

Maintenance Phase Treatment

The maintenance phase of drug therapy is aimed at preventing recurrence of episodes of BD. Interestingly there are no novel maintenance drugs but actually the same ones used in the acute phase of therapy. There is little evidence that these drugs work as well in preventing relapses in young people as they do in adults. The maintenance phase usually lasts from one to two years. This depends to a degree on the level of impairment, the chronicity of the condition, the number of episodes of bipolarity, and the level of stability reached by the youth and the environment in which she lives. While most young patients are able to get off these medications, there will be times that this will prove impossible. Sometimes relapse follows quickly upon stopping the medications. As with some adults, a decision will be made that drug therapy will be maintained indefinitely to help the child or adolescent progress in life, socially, educationally, and vocationally without the risk of further decompensation.

What are the Drugs?

Below is a list of the major mood stabilizers. Of all of these, Lithium, Depakote, and Tegretol are the three most commonly used.

LITHIUM—Approved for children 12 years and older.
DEPAKOTE—Approved for children 2 years and older for seizures.
TEGRETOL—Approved for all ages for seizures.
GABAPENTIN—Approved for young people 18 and older. Approved only for epilepsy.
LAMICTAL—Approved for young people 18 and older. Approved for seizures in children.
TOPAMAX—Approved for young people 18 and older. Approved for seizures.
TRILEPTAL—Approved for children 4 and older. Approved for seizures.

LITHIUM

The most well-known, well-studied, and longest used drug for BD, Lithium has been popularized through the many stories told by sufferers from all walks of life. Despite the mostly favorable publicity, the misconception exists that it's for very sick people and can be dangerous. In fact, no evidence exists that people who take Lithium are any sicker than those on other medications. The fear of Lithium generally springs from the well-publicized stories of the quite rare Lithium toxicity reaction. I have prescribed Lithium to many hundreds of patients, young and old, and have only witnessed this reaction once. As usual, the horror stories predominate and overshadow the essentially safe and ameliorative effects of this drug. People can and do take Lithium for years with only positive results.

Doctors prescribe Lithium off label for children under twelve years old but as true BD is rarely diagnosed under that age most of the prescribing is done for teenagers. I have prescribed Lithium, although rarely, to outpatients younger than twelve years old as a first choice drug. I have also monitored its use in discharged patients who started on Lithium while hospitalized for a severe psychiatric state. I have seen no negative effects. In addition to the rarity of true BD in young children another reason that it is not commonly given is that the required blood tests to monitor Lithium levels can frighten young children. Additionally, fewer studies have been done on very young children using Lithium as compared to the studies done on teenagers. Still, anecdotal evidence strongly favors its use with little fear of negative effects. Since there has been more study in young children using Antipsychotic use, I prefer to start with a drug from that category. After failure in that category I then turn to Lithium in the young group, as an augmenter or as monotherapy. With teenagers I use Lithium more freely and to great advantage.

Side Effects of Lithium

The side effects of Lithium are usually quite mild and tolerable. It is not uncommon to experience increased thirst, increased urination, headache, drowsiness, a mild tremor of the hand, itching, mild elevation of white blood cells, thinning of hair and skin, mild nausea, and a general feeling of uneasiness in the body. Additionally, Lithium sometimes can harm the thyroid gland and kidney over the long term, even when correct dosing is given, so it's essential that kidney and thyroid function tests be done regularly when your child takes this drug. Before beginning Lithium, your child should have a complete blood count, an ECG, and thyroid and kidney tests. Most of the mild side effects pass as one becomes used to the drug.

Lithium toxicity differs dramatically from these side effects. As treatment begins, your psychiatrist will monitor Lithium blood levels ensuring that your child's dose never goes high enough to cause toxicity. This essential blood testing makes Lithium a safe drug. In the event Lithium blood levels are not monitored, toxicity is a risk. The symptoms usually include:

- Confusion
- Drowsiness
- Twitching
- Loss of coordination
- Muscle weakness
- Severe nausea and diarrhea
- Slurred speech
- Visual changes
- Vomiting
- Loss of consciousness
- Abnormal muscle movements
- Convulsions
- Rarely coma and death can occur

Lithium toxicity is a medical emergency and usually treated in a hospital where bloods can be monitored and blood dialysis performed if necessary.

How Lithium is Used

Lithium carbonate is given orally. I usually administer Lithium starting with the regular Lithium 300 mgs tablets. After several days of that dose I increase it for a few days. By the end of a week I send for a Lithium blood level. I am aiming at a Lithium level of between .4 meq/l to 1.0 meq/l. The ideal level is usually considered about .6-.75meq/l. I will raise the dose to 900 or 1200 if needed and monitor the clinical response and again get a Lithium blood level every week for the first 3–4 weeks. After stabilization—when the mood and blood levels are both steady—I can reduce the testing to every few months.

Before starting your child on Lithium, your psychiatrist will take a complete history of any medical conditions. He will advise you to maintain your youngster's regular salt intake and will order a complete blood count, kidney and thyroid blood tests, and an ECG.

TABLE 12
COMMON LITHIUM PREPARATIONS

BRAND NAME	GENERIC NAME	AVAILABLE DOASAGES (MGS)
ESKALITH	LITHIUM CARBONATE	300
ESKALITH CR	LITHIUM CARBONATE CONTROLLED RELEASE	450
LITHOBID	LITHIUM CARBONATE EXTENDED RELEASE	300

TEGRETOL (Carbamazine) is an antiepileptic drug used commonly for BD in adults and young people. It is not approved for use in BD and is given off label. It is approved for use in epilepsy for children as well as adults. Despite this off label use, it has been reported as quite successful in some of the few trials reported. The dosage recommended for young people is up to 300 mgs a day.

Side Effects of Tegretol

The most common side effects of Tegretol are dizziness, drowsiness, nausea, vomiting, and unsteadiness. Although there is sometimes a transient lowering of the white blood cell count, which reverses, there is some danger of more severe blood disorders such as bone marrow depression with lowering of white blood cells and platelets or severe skin reactions such as toxic epidermal necrolysis and Stevens Johnson syndrome, which are highly dangerous, although rare. Liver function is sometimes compromised as well.

Before prescribing Tegretol a complete history and physical examination is necessary. There should be a complete examination of the skin as well as a complete blood count and other blood tests to be sure of the level of liver function.

TABLE 1 3
TEGRETOL PREPARATIONS

BRAND NAME	GENERIC NAME	AVAILABLE DOSAGES (MGS)
TEGRETOL	CARBAMAZEPINE	100, 200
TEGRETOL XR	CARBAMAZEPINE	100, 200, 400
TEGRETOL SYRUP	CARBAMEZEPINE	100 MGS/5ML

VALPROIC ACID (DIVALPROATE)—Also known as Depakote, Depakote ER, and Depakene

DEPAKOTE, as it is most well-known, is another anti-epileptic medication used as a mood stabilizer. Like with other antiepileptics this medication is used off label in young people. But it is widely used and considered almost as good as Lithium for BD. It is specifically used quite a bit in teenagers with BD with good results. As mentioned above, it is sometimes used as a first line monotherapy like Lithium or in combination with other drugs.

Side Effects of Valproic Acid

Like the other medications, there are occasionally side effects with this drug including drowsiness, dizziness, nausea, vomiting, weight gain, itching and rash, and mild tremor. More serious side effects include decreased platelet functioning, decreased ability to form clots, liver malfunction, and even rarely pancreatitis. In young females it can cause an increase in testosterone causing Polycystic Ovarian Syndrome (PCOS) with eggs in the ovary turning into cysts (often reversible). Additionally, it can cause fetal abnormalities such as spina bifida. It should not be used in young people who have urea cycle abnormalities.

Before starting this drug a complete medical history and physical exam is necessary. There should also be a complete blood count, clotting tests, tests of kidney function, urine analysis, and a pregnancy test for girls. Caution should be taken and full disclosure about PCOS and pregnancy issues should be made.

TABLE 14
COMMON VALRPOIC ACID PREPARATIONS

BRAND NAME	GENERIC NAME	AVAILABLE DOSAGES (MGS)
DEPAKOTE	DIVALPROEX SPDIUM	125, 250, 500
DEPAKOTE ER	DIVALPROEX SODIUM	250, 500
DEPAKOTE SPRINKLES	DIVALPROEX SODIUM	125
DEPAKENE	VALPROIC ACID	250
DEPAKOTE SYRUP	VALRPOIC ACID	250 AND 500 MGS/5ML

Other Uses of Mood Stabilizers in Children and Adolescents
Mood stabilizers have been useful in the following conditions:

- Aggressive behavior disorders such as Conduct Disorder
- High activity disorders such as ADHD
- Intermittent Explosive Disorder
- Other behavior disorders that have not responded to other medications

CHAPTER SEVEN

TREATMENT OF ANXIETY DISORDERS

"Josh was always a lot more sensitive than his sisters. When he was a toddler he was more affected by things like loud noises, meeting new people and our going out at night and leaving him with a sitter. Now he's in his second year at preschool and he's started trying to avoid going. It's become a terrible problem each morning with screaming, tantrums, and fighting until we give in and let him stay home."

"Mary has always wanted to do well at everything she tried. We used to tell her to calm down and enjoy but she always wanted to be the best at everything. Now her third grade teacher tells us she is very hard on herself at school academically and even in gym. And at home she's always worried about something and never relaxes. We worry she'll never be able to enjoy life."

"My daughter Sharon is fifteen and came home the other day looking pale. She said she was talking to her friends in the cafeteria and started to feel unreal, nervous, and thought she was going to die. She said she started to have trouble breathing, felt the walls were closing in on her, and she had to run out of the school. Since then she has become panicky at home as well. She worries constantly that this will happen again and refuses to leave the house since she is scared she might need help somewhere and not be able to get it."

Anxiety disorders like those described above—school phobia in the first, generalized anxiety disorder in the second, and panic disorder with agoraphobia in the third—are the most common mental disorders in young people. Estimates of their prevalence range from 10 to 20 percent of youngsters under eighteen years of age, a remarkably large number. Not only is the prevalence high, but only a small fraction of these children receive proper treatment and the results of these disorders going untreated can be devastating. It has been reported that the incidence of many mental disorders occurring later in life increases if earlier childhood and adolescent anxiety disorders are left untreated. These include serious adult depressive and anxiety disorders, suicidal tendencies, mental breakdowns, school failure, academic and work failure, and substance abuse.

What is the Difference Between Fear and Anxiety?

Every child—and every adult—has fears. Without fear we would unable to develop. We would be unaware of many dangers that exist in the world, things which could hurt us. Fear is a rational, appropriate response to danger. As we get older, we learn more and more about threats and develop the capacity and confidence to handle our fears, so we begin to overcome them. The younger we are, the more fearful we are, and the more global are our responses.

Common childhood fears include:

Separation from caretakers
New situations
The dark
Loud noises including thunderstorms
Monsters
Getting lost or abducted
Animals, especially dogs, snakes, and insects

A parent dying
The many new challenges that accompany normal development, such as the first day of school, a first date

Many childhood fears seem irrational to us, but if we think about it, we realize that without the experience of living and growing, childhood fears are not irrational at all. No one ever completely lives without fear. While there is a wide variation in how each of us responds to fear, it is always present.

Anxiety resembles, but is different from, fear. It is essentially an irrational fear based on inner—psychological—issues. Sometimes it presents as what appears to be a prolongation of common childhood fears, as with a ten-year-old who fears the dark excessively or a seven-year-old who cannot separate from his parents and go to school. These prolongations are no longer simple fears of childhood but are probably symptoms of one of the anxiety disorders: a diagnosable mental disorder. Since many anxiety symptoms resemble the normal fears of childhood we often mistakenly say that such sufferers seem immature or infantile, while in fact they are suffering from an anxiety disorder. Anxiety sometimes feels like worry, apprehension, excessive shyness, all the way to fear of everyday situations and even panic. Often there are physical symptoms like a racing heart, trouble breathing, sweating, dizziness, headache, nausea, vomiting and diarrhea, and occasionally, muscle spasms. Sometimes there is a sensation of finger-tingling and weakness in the muscles of the legs and arms. Occasionally children will pass out as a result of anxiety. In addition, while anxious, most children have trouble functioning well in school and at home. They have difficulty learning and socializing. Very anxious children misperceive and often exaggerate environmental dangers leading to avoidance of many situations—this is called a phobia. Over all, most children suffering from ongoing anxiety eventually lose confidence, feel helpless and vulnerable, and develop depression.

Causes of Anxiety

We are not certain as to the cause of anxiety disorders, but mental health practitioners have always felt that buried inner conflicts often have to do with these disorders. Thus, causes include the following:

- An inner conflict between such feelings as dependency and anger at important figures is a common generator of anxiety states.
- Excessive trauma, such as child physical or sexual abuse, might give rise to persistent anxiety states.
- Some anxiety disorders are thought to have a significant basis in genetic inheritance, such as obsessive compulsive disorder and panic disorder.
- Some anxiety symptoms are learned through observation of family members who suffer from such problems—learned anxiety.
- Some have considered abnormal neurotransmitter activity as a cause.
- Some medical conditions occasionally give rise to excessive anxiety, such as hyperthyroidism, certain tumors, some neurological illnesses, heart rhythm and valve disorders, certain lung diseases especially with shortness of breath, and some infections.
- Some medications cause anxiety as a side effect.

WHICH ANXIETY DISORDERS APPEAR IN YOUNG PEOPLE?

The anxiety disorders are those mental disorders with anxiety, in some form, as the major symptom. It should be noted that anxiety is present in nearly all people who suffer from any mental disorder but is the main symptom in these disorders. Anxiety disorders have been categorized by the way the anxiety manifests itself for the most part. The following are the main types. Many of the disorders overlap as well.

1. **Separation Anxiety Disorder** (SAD) - This disorder's main characteristic is anxiety when a child leaves home or people to whom she is attached. While separation fear is common and expected in young children, especially during the first and second years of life, it usually abates as a child approaches the school years to the point that separation anxiety is not present. SAD has the following symptoms:

A serious worry that something bad (often including death) will happen to parents or caregivers upon separation *or* to the child, upon separation from the parents or caregivers. This anxiety is manifested even when a separation is anticipated

Worries over abduction or being kidnapped

School refusal in order to stay near parent, often accompanied by stomachache and headache complaints around separation time

Fear of being alone or even going to sleep without the parent

Bad dreams about separation

Bed wetting

Rage episodes and tantrums and begging not to be forced to separate

As mentioned above, while we don't know the exact mechanism of how an anxiety disorder like SAD is generated, the disorder often appears after a major separation, a move to new surroundings, loss of an important care-taking figure, in a house with over protective parents, and in families with others who have the same condition.

2. **Generalized Anxiety Disorder** (GAD) - This disorder is characterized by excessive worrying. It is hard to specify the source of worry since it varies quite a bit and is general in nature. The child often feels on edge and is tense most of the time. As a result she is often tired, has muscular tension states, and finds it difficult to relax, concentrate, or just let loose. There is irritation and often trouble sleeping as well. Often such children are quite perfectionistic and come from homes which are pressure cookers for performance.

3. **Panic Attacks and Panic Disorder** (with or without agoraphobia) - **A Panic Attack** is one of the most uncomfortable symptoms known to us. Sometimes called anxiety attacks, panic attacks are a discreet period of time during which a child or teenager feels intense fear, often of doom, going crazy, dying, or some vague dread of being out control. They can last anywhere from several minutes to a half hour. There is an intense need to escape. An outpouring of adrenaline leads to many physical symptoms along with ideas of death or going crazy. The following are listed as the most common symptoms:

Shortness of breath
Choking feeling
Racing pounding heart, sweating, trembling, chills, or hot flushes
Chest discomfort
Nausea and abdominal distress
Feeling unreal or perceiving the world as unreal
Dizziness, feeling like fainting or in fact fainting
Tingling or numbness in the extremities

Panic Disorder occurs when a worry is experienced after one or more panic attacks and the child begins to anticipate another and as a result often alters his behavior to avoid being unable to escape or get help if one might occur. Thus many children develop an avoidant (phobic) lifestyle to avoid such situations as leaving home, crowds, being on a bridge, and public transportation. This syndrome is called *agoraphobia* from the Greek word *agora* meaning marketplace referring to an open place. Some people never develop the agoraphobia but simply have *panic disorder* with recurrent panic attacks and worry, but no avoidance.

4. **Obsessive Compulsive Disorder** (OCD) - This anxiety disorder is characterized by the presence obsessions and compulsions. **Obessions** are, unwanted irrational persistent thoughts, mental pictures or ideas and urges which cause great anxiety. Sometimes there are persistent unanswerable questions, such as "Why is the world here?" or "Why does a chair have four and not three legs?" which can plague a child for many hours. Most often the obsessive thoughts have to do with germ contamination, dirt, doubts, fear of doing violent or aggressive or sexual acts, or worries about illness. These intrusive and troubling thoughts, although they might not seem that way, are in fact usually perceived as irrational by the youngster. Although great attempts are made to suppress them, the obsessions come back to plague the victim with great anxiety after a period of time.

Compulsions are repetitive behaviors associated with obsessions such as hand washing, ordering things just so, or checking to make sure that ovens and lights are off again and again to ward off perceived disorder and danger. Praying, locking things over and over, and repeating words or phrases or counting are also common. Those with compulsions also may have the need to do things an even number of times with each hand, to take a certain number of steps, or to have things "just perfect" before taking actions. The whole picture comes to resemble great superstition but is simply the attempt to ward off the dangers lurking in the obsessive mind. The OCD syndrome is a source of great distress and sometimes leads to paralysis and despair.

5. **Social Phobia** - This painful syndrome is characterized by excessive anxiety related to social events or performance situations where there is the fear of exposure or scrutiny by others. There is a fear of anxiety or even panic which would secondarily lead to humiliation or disgrace. The fear can be quite specific such as speaking in class, or become more general where it can lead to widespread avoidance to areas like socializing, group situations, or even speaking to people at school like teachers or friends. It can be quite disabling. In children who have excessive social anxiety it can present as fearfulness with any stranger, having to cling to a parent, or signs of distress in social situations like crying, tantrums, or freezing up.

6. **Selective Mutism** - This syndrome is considered to be a severe example of social phobia where the child presents as failing to speak in certain social situations where there is such an expectation such as in school or sometimes simply outside the house. There is full ability to speak and often a child can be heard speaking well and loudly to a parent (such as in the waiting room of my office only to go mute upon entering my consulting room). This diagnosis is made after other psychiatric syndromes are ruled out which might interfere with speaking such as autism or language/speech/communication disorders.

7. **Post Traumatic Stress Disorder** (PTSD) - This anxiety disorder occurs after a young person is victim of, or exposed to, or a witness to a traumatic event(s) in which there is the experience of perceived possibility of death and/or bodily injury, and during

which there was great fear, helplessness, horror, mental disorganization, or agitation. This can be one event (major car accident) or a series such as repeated sexual or physical abuse. PTSD can occur rather soon after a trauma or actually appear many months later. This syndrome is particularly common in children in the foster population who have been neglected and abused. Many of the behavioral problems they manifest are due to traumatic anxiety they are experiencing.

As a result of the event(s) there is:

An ongoing re-experiencing of the event(s) through mental images, thoughts, or perceptions of it

Repetitive play involving aspects of the trauma (violent play themes over and over)

Repetitive nightmares

Repetitive re-enactments of the event

Dissociative flashbacks (during which the person feels as if he is re-experiencing the event, hallucinates, and misperceives events)

Severe anxiety and altered physiology (startle response) when exposed to cues reminiscent of the trauma

Avoidance of anything which reminds one of the event

Altered memory

Feeling distant and estranged

A narrowing of feeling experience

An attitude which conveys a feeling of having a foreshortened future

Sleep problems, irritability, worry, startle response, trouble concentrating, hypervigilence, excessive anger.

8. **Specific Phobia** – A phobia is a marked and repetitive fear which is stimulated by a situation or object. It is unreasonable, irrational, and is usually recognized as such except in younger children. When exposed to the phobic stimulus there can be great anxiety, possibly a panic attack, crying, a frozen look, tantrums, and excessive clinging. There are literally thousands of phobias described but the more common ones are of animals, storms, heights, blood, medical procedures, elevators, airplanes, tunnels, insects, or getting an injury.

The anxiety disorders listed above do not always occur in isolation. In fact, there is quite a bit of overlap. It is well known that there is a high degree of overlap of Separation Anxiety Disorder, Generalized Anxiety Disorder, and Social Phobia with as much as a 40 percent overlap of symptomology.

TREATMENT OF ANXIETY DISORDERS WITH PSYCHOTROPIC MEDICATION

Therapy First

Any young person suffering from an anxiety disorder should receive a full evaluation after which a trial of *some form of psychotherapy* (see chapter on therapies) is tried before making the step to medication. The form of therapy is usually multimodal including, possibly in some combination:

Family therapy
Individual dynamic therapy
Parent education
Behavior therapy
Work with school personnel
Parent-child therapy

MEDICATION

In general the best medications to use to treat anxiety disorders are the *antidepressant drugs.* These medications have been discussed in another chapter of this book. Although there is little empirical proof of the use of these medications for anxiety disorders, information about them is extrapolated from adult studies.

Antidepressants for Anxiety Disorders

The ***SSRI antidepressant medications*** are considered the best choice at this time. For OCD Zoloft, Prozac, Luvox and Paxil have gotten good results. TCA (tricyclic) antidepressants have also been used for OCD with Anafranil being quite successful. For reasons mentioned in the chapter on antidepressants, I prefer the use of SSRI's over TCA's. For Generalized Anxiety, Separation Anxiety, Social Phobia, Specific Phobias, PTSD and Selective Mutism, SSRI antidepressants are the first drugs of choice. For Panic Disorder SSRI's are, again, the first choice, but TCA's have also been successful. If anxiety is very severe to the point of leading to disorganization—a psychiatric term that basically means the blurring of the ability to perceive reality—use of antipsychotic medication (discussed elsewhere) is justified. It must be remembered that antidepressants take at least a few weeks to work and do not quell acute anxiety. Over time they will help in preventing almost all anxiety symptoms.

What about the Common Benzodiazepines for Anxiety Disorders?

The benzodiazepines are extremely common in adult psychiatry. They are also called tranquilizers or anxiolytic drugs. These drugs immediately relieve anxiety and insomnia. *There is, however, little evidence for their successful use in people under eighteen years of age other than for sedation prior to surgery or medical procedures and occasionally in treating very severe and disabling anxiety symptoms on a very short term basis.* These medications are approved for psychiatric use in adults and are used off label by psychiatrists for younger people.

The mode of action of benzodiazepines in the central nervous system is thought to be mostly involved with the neurotransmitter called GABA (gamma amino butyric acid). These medications increase the availability of GABA which in turn slows the transmission of nerve impulses throughout the body. In the central nervous system there are thought to be two receptors for these medications that in turn produce anxiety relief and sedation. In general, these medications have been used to treat insomnia, control anxiety, prevent muscle spasms, and as anti-seizure drugs in adults. They induce calmness and relaxation and decrease tension. These meds also have side effects including:

Motor coordination problems
Drowsiness, tiredness
Nausea
Dry mouth
Diarrhea and constipation
Tremors, slurred speech, trouble thinking clearly, confusion, dizziness and difficulty remembering, coordination difficulties, disorientation

Mood instability with cases of manic-like euphoria as well as depression
Paradoxical anxiety and hostility

These medications have a moderate rate of substance abuse as well, which was discovered in the 1980's after about twenty years of being used to treat anxiety. Thus, these drugs are considered possible subjects of abuse and addiction and are controlled in most states. Benzodiazepine abuse becomes common in mid to late adolescence. Abuse of these drugs is highest among people who are addicted to other drugs such as alcohol, heroin, and cocaine. There is an addiction syndrome with increasing tolerance of the medication so that a person needs more and more of it to produce the desired effect (a high) and a withdrawal syndrome if stopped including:

- Anxiety, agitation, panic, and terror
- Insomnia, nightmares
- Dizziness, dry mouth, muscle cramps
- Feeling ill like with the flu
- Difficulties with memory and concentration
- Headache, fatigue, and weakness
- Overall increased sensitivity to sound, touch, and light
- Dilated pupils
- Body aches and pains
- Hallucinations
- Suspiciousness, depression, and feeling unreal
- Hot flushes
- Nausea, high heart rate, and hypertension
- Tremor
- Convulsions, coma, and violence, if withdrawal is rapid

If withdrawal progresses, patients often find that their physical and mental health improves and they report better mood and cognition.

Benzodiazepines are divided into short and long acting types. Basically, the short acting variety are best for anxiety and are eliminated quickly, which cuts down on daytime sedation (hangover). The downside is that they cause a greater craving, as their blood concentrations fall off quickly, which also causes a sharper withdrawal syndrome. The longer acting medications are better for sleep, but can cause the common side effect of daytime sedation. Both types induce sleep quite well if treating insomnia, but the longer acting ones might keep someone asleep longer. Examples of the types are:

TABLE 15
SHORT ACTING BENZODIAZEPINES

TRADE NAME	GENERIC NAME	AVAILABLE DOSAGES (MGS)
XANAX	ALPRAZOLAM	.25, .5, 1, 2
LORAZEPAM	ATIVAN	.5, 1, 2
HALCION	TRIAZOLAM	.125, .5
ESTAZOLAM	PROSOM	1, 2

TABLE 16
MID AND LONG ACTING BENZODIAZEPINES

BRAND NAME	GENERIC NAME	AVAILABLE DOSAGES (MGS)
LIBRIUM	LIBRIUM	5, 10, 25 MGS
VALIUM	DIAZEPAM	2, 5, 10 MGS
KLONOPIN	CLONAZEPAM	.5, 1, AND 2 MGS
TRANXENE	CLORAZEPATE	3.75. 7.5, AND 15 MGS
DALMANE	FLURAZEPAM	15 AND 30 MGS
RESTORIL	TEMAZEPAM	7.5, 15, 22.5, AND 30 MGS

Other Medications for Anxiety in Children and Teenagers

1. ANTIHISTAMINES

These medications are usually used to combat allergies. They also have been used as sedatives. The onset of the sedation is rather quick. The compounds decrease the effect of the neurotransmitter *histamine* which causes arousal. These medications are less effective than other anti-anxiety medications and sometimes the dose has to be raised to the point that side effects might occur including:

Drowsiness
Dry mouth
Constipation
Rapid heart rate
Problems with coordination, weakness, and concentration.

TABLE 17
COMMON ANTIHISTAMINES

BRAND NAME	GENERIC NAME	AVAILABLE DOSAGES (MGS)
ATARAX/VISTARIL	HYDROXYZINE	10, 25, 50 MGS
BENADRYL	DIPHENHYDRAMINE	10, 25, 50 MGS

2. **BUSPAR** (Buspirone) is another medication used for anxiety. It is unrelated to the benzodiazepines. It is thought to act by increasing availability of Serotonin. It takes a few weeks to work. It does not cause sedation and is thought to be quite effective against some of the bodily symptoms of anxiety such as intestinal and cardiovascular symptoms. There is no substance abuse potential. Side effects are usually mild and include nausea, dizziness and headaches. It comes in strengths of 5, 10, 15, and 20 mgs.

3. **ANTIPSYCHOTIC MEDICATION** is very rarely used for children with severe anxiety disorders. These are discussed in a separate chapter.

4. **BETA BLOCKERS** block the effects of the sympathetic nervous system (they decrease the sensitivity of the so-called beta receptors in the sympathetic nervous system). In addition to being used to treat anxiety, they are widely used to treat many disorders such as heart failure hypertension, angina, hyperthyroidism, migraines, and many other conditions. They block the effects of norepinepherine. They are not addictive. They are most effective against the physical effects of anxiety such as tremor, trembling, blushing, tension, increased heart rate, shaky voice, and high blood pressure. They are especially good when used for stage fright. *Inderal* (propanalol) is the most commonly used beta blocker in psychiatry. It comes in 10, 20, 40, 60, and 80 mg pills.

CHAPTER 8

SLEEP DISORDERS AND MEDICATION

"Our son Randy has always been a hyper-type but over the years he has received great school treatment and understanding. He was diagnosed as having ADD and has done well with tutoring and special programs. But he has never slept well and I read that his poor sleep can lead to all sorts of problems."

"Joannie has been a poor sleeper all of her life but when she turned seven last year it got even worse. She goes to sleep late, wakes up a lot, and is always tired. I work two jobs and its exhausting me too. What can I do?"

"Sandy has been scaring us. She seems to wake up screaming, terrified, and agitated. She bolts up. After a few minutes she goes back to sleep. It not only scares us but she doesn't even remember the whole thing the next morning."

In general the use of medication for common sleep problems for children and teenagers should be a last resort. Most parents who complain of sleep problems in their children can, if guided by their common sense, pediatricians or others, solve the problem through the appropriate use of bed time preparation or other interventions. While the use of sleeping pills (hypnotic medication) has grown astronomically in adults this should not take place for our youth.

Unfortunately there has been a rise in prescription medication for childhood and teenage sleep problems in our country. In some cases, such as children with psychiatric problems, sleep problems are part of the syndrome and the treatment of the problem correctly should restore normal sleep. In other cases there are types of sleep problems which are of organic biological origin which might need an appropriate medication such as sleepwalking, bedwetting, or night terrors (like Sandy). But for children and teenagers as a whole the use of medication should be withheld until all other interventions have been found not to work.

What should we expect about sleep?

In general some sleep knowledge is helpful. Children sleep less as they get older. Newborns and infants can spend half of their time sleeping. But by four months old, regularity of sleep starts with the establishment of regular circadian patterns. These regular biological patterns contribute to regularities in sleep and waking, activity levels, hormone secretion, and other biological phenomena. Although four months marks the establishment of some regularity of sleep cycles it is not usually until one year old that the frequency of night awakenings significantly diminishes. By four years old most children do not need to nap but often do need eleven to twelve hours of sleep. By early to mid-adolescence sleep patterns are quite close to those of adults who require about seven to eight hours of sleep.

Sleep problems

It should be noted that so-called sleep problems have a lot to do with what particular parents find tolerable in their children which in turn is affected by their own sleep patterns, the subculture in which a child is raised, and the overall tolerance of the household to a child's awakenings. It is also important for parents to know what to expect at various ages in order to know when a sleep problem exists.

It is important that a child gets enough sleep. A child who does not get enough sleep can be plagued by many problems which include:

Irritability
Impulsivity
Inattention
Moodiness
Aggressiveness
Fatigue
Learning problems
Child/parent interaction disturbances
Overweight
Having to be awakened regularly

In addition to the common causes of insomnia including stress, anxiety, stimulus overload, and caffeine, there are other causes which should be ruled out such as obstructive sleep apnea, restless leg syndrome, side effects of medication including ADHD and antidepressant medications, chronic illness, autism, developmental delays, ADHD itself, depression, and anxiety disorders. After these have been ruled out, common insomnia can be handled without the use of special sleep medications in almost all cases.

Sleep Hygiene

It is important and often tedious for parents to do what is necessary to ensure that their child sleeps well and enough. Nearly all common behavioral sleep problems, such as bed time refusal, bed time resistance, difficulty falling asleep, frequent awakenings, getting up too early, and the like can be overcome without the use of medication. Most important in accomplishing this is the practice of what has been called sleep hygiene which in essence contains the following characteristics:

Make sure that a regular bed time (and wake time) is adhered to and that any bed time rituals start thirty minutes before the desired sleep time
Bed time rituals should include pleasant activities such as reading to your child, rubbing, and soothing
Sleep onset associations like being rocked or fed by you at the time of going to sleep should not include the parent as much as possible—for example, try to put the child in bed before falling asleep when rocking
Make sure that daily schedules are adhered to in all areas of life
Limit napping
Make sure your child has a balanced diet with enough food
Make sure your child gets adequate amounts of exercise
Make sure that your child is protected from excessive chaos in the house such as violence, shouting, emotional upheavals, and quarreling.
Bed time should be after three to four hours after eating
There should be no heavy exercise for at least two hours
The bedroom should be of normal temperature
After dinner the atmosphere should be one of relaxation and quiet activities
Emotional issues should be avoided as should any rough play and caffeine.
Try to help child resolve emotional issues during day and not before sleep
The room should be dark and quiet without clocks or televisions
Teach your child some relaxation techniques such as deep breathing

The major thing to keep in mind is that as sleep time approaches the goal is to induce a relaxed drowsiness, not an emotional or active time.

If a parent abides by these sleep hygiene suggestions the great majority of children will sleep well consistently. Of course from time to time there will be awakenings, especially if a child is sick, disturbed, or scared, but these are episodic and usually respond to gentle and firm reassurances and do not require special interventions. And do remember that not all children sleep exactly the same and there will be variation from child to child. But knowing your child's natural patterns and adjusting your ways to your child's rhythms go a long way to pleasant nighttimes.

What about kids with psychiatric problems?

A child and adolescent psychiatrist sees many children with mental disorders whose parents complain that their child has trouble falling asleep, in addition to their other problems.
Specifically the following psychiatric disorders have associated sleep problems:

1. ADHD—many children who have ADHD have trouble sleeping because of impulsivity and hyperactivity and sometimes because the side effects of stimulant medication, especially if taken late in the day, can cause insomnia. Clonidine or an antihistamine (see below) is often used in these children as one of the outstanding side effects of these medications is fatigue/drowsiness and sleepiness. Clonidine is often used in the daytime as well, as an adjunctive medication to the stimulant meds used in treating ADHD. When used in the day for ADHD, there is now an increasingly extended release form.

2. Anxiety states—especially separation anxiety—often cause sleeplessness. Also worrying too much and the general inability to relax found in anxious children. Treatment of the anxiety state with some form of psychotherapy as well use of one of SSRI antidepressant medications will help with the insomnia. Occasionally an SSRI might cause insomnia as well, especially if taken late in the day.

3. Depressive disorders often include sleep problems. Not only insomnia but also hypersomnia (especially in adolescents) is a common symptom. Treatment of the depressive disorder itself should relieve the sleep symptoms.

4. Children with Pervasive Developmental Disorders (Autism) and Mental Retardation often have trouble sleeping. In addition to behavioral therapy these children often do well with an antihistamine such as Benadryl. The use of Melatonin is also used in this population. This is a hormone produced in the brain and has been associated with the sleep cycle. Although it has never been scientifically shown to increase sleep it is sold over the counter to many people. It has side effects, including depression, fatigue, blood pressure variability, and possibly fertility problems amongst others, and the manufacture of it is uncontrolled by the government. Thus doses could be wrong and blood levels could increase to high levels. I have never suggested that children take this medication in light of the unproven efficacy, uncontrolled manufacturing, and possible deleterious side effects.

5. Children with Post Traumatic Stress Disorder have many sleepless nights due to bad dreams and even flashbacks at night. These children have been traumatized by an event and the reestablishment of equilibrium will take time and care

to be restored. Treatment of PTSD should go a long way to diminishing this problem. If the anxiety associated with PTSD is crippling, then in addition to an SSRI, a sleeping medication might be given short term (see below for sleep meds).

6. In teenagers we often see the onset of insomnia occur with the use of illicit drugs especially alcohol, stimulants, cocaine, and party drugs which can cause great anxiety and agitation.

Certain Medications and Illnesses

Certain medication such as cold medications, steroids, asthma drugs, thyroid hormone and diet pills can cause sleeplessness. You should check with your pediatrician to be sure that nothing your child takes might be causing insomnia.

Any illness and especially ones with pain involved often result in trouble sleeping as well. Of course proper medical treatment will help but sometimes a sleeping medication is needed until the problem remits.

OTHER SLEEP DISORDERS AND THEIR TREATMENT

There are a group of sleep disorders called **Parasomnias**. These syndromes present as unusual behaviors or movements that occur during sleep. They occur mostly in children and are rarely serious. They usually are gone by adolescence and the most effective interventions are parent education and counseling. Medication is rarely needed for most cases. They are rarely associated with major mental disorders. The most common ones encountered in practice are Nightmares, Night Terrors, Sleepwalking, and Bedwetting.

Nightmares

Nightmares or bad dreams are quite common in young people. These are dreams in which the child experiences himself in danger, vulnerable, frightened, and helpless. There is great distress, sometimes even panic and horror. Common themes often involve being chased, drowning, and other frightening losses of control. These dreams usually happen in the second part of the night and the child often wakes up scared and remembers the dream content. The child is often quite anxious, possibly believing that the dream was reality. He has a fast heart rate and might be perspiring as well. Children usually need soothing and reassurance. Sometimes from the content of the nightmare the parent will be able to figure out what might be causing a passing stress or anxiety and might be able to help. Of course there might be causes for repetitive nightmares such as chronic stress/anxiety. Some physiological causes might be the administration of certain antidepressants or stimulant medication for ADHD and post traumatic stress disorder. If nightmares have become disruptive to the point of interfering with functioning then treatment to decrease stress, a fitness program, relaxation therapy, yoga, and even meditation have all been reported to help. In the most severe cases, such as those following a severe stressor, medication has been used with success and includes: the antidepressants Trazadone or Serzone, some mood stabilizer, and possibly a Benzodiazepine anti-anxiety drug for the short term (a week or so).

Night Terror Disorder (Pavor Nocturnus)

This is frightening event to those who witness it. Typically the child bolts upright from sleep with eyes wide open (although often not able to recognize family members), appears frightened often to the point of panic, and is screaming, confused, and inconsolable. The heart rate is elevated, there is shortness of breath, and he might be sweating as well. There is what appears to be acute terrifying distress. The child usually cannot be awakened. The episode usually occurs in the first third of the night and he falls right back to sleep. There is amnesia for the event the next morning. Although this is a dramatic event it is not particularly serious in the long term. It occurs rarely and usually disappears by teenage years. Some hypothesized causes are fatigue, new environments, fever, obstructive sleep apnea, and stress of some sort. As with nightmares the way to handle this is to be reassuring and comforting and not to panic yourself. Practicing good sleep hygiene is a parent's best bet. If they become frequent and/or disrupt family life the use of benzodiazepines for a short amount of time has been found helpful. Some parents have reported that 1–5 hydoxytryptophan which is sold over the counter and metabolized to become serotonin in the body has allayed these terror attacks.

Somnambulism (Sleepwalking)

This parasomnia is characterized by a child getting up and walking around. Eyes are open but responsiveness is either absent or inappropriate. Walking around can vary from quiet walking to agitated running. There is usually a glassy dazed stare. Sometimes the child can go to the bathroom or engage in other activities. Rarely there is violence. There is amnesia for the event. After the episode the child can be found sleeping somewhere in the house. There appears to be a genetic contribution to causation. Additionally, sleep deprivation, a chaotic environment, stress, some sleeping pills, and antipsychotic drugs, stimulants, or antihistamines might cause these episodes. It is also associated with PTSD, panic disorder, and possibly dissociative identity disorder. Some medical conditions including gastro esophageal reflux, fever, asthma, and obstructive sleep apnea are present. As in other parasomnias treatment becomes necessary if there is resultant family disturbance or increased frequency. Since children can hurt themselves by accidents such as falling down stairs or getting outside the house, safety measures have to be taken such as trying to make the first floor of a house the sleeping location, locking doors and windows, clearing obstructions, putting heavy drapes over glass windows, and possibly setting an alarm which will sound if the child gets out of bed. Treatment consists of clearing up any associated medical condition and rarely the use of medication including the short term benzodiapine Klonopin or Trazadone.

Enuresis (Bedwetting)

Some consider this another parasomnia since one type occurs at night—nocturnal enuresis. The other type is daytime wetting called diurnal enuresis. Here we are only concerned with the former. This is usually called bedwetting and is the involuntary voiding of urine while asleep after the time bladder control should have occurred (4–5 years old). Primary enuresis is that type that occurs when a child has never had a dry period while the secondary type is after having achieved dryness (at least six months and is usually due to a stress or a medical illness).

Bedwetting runs in families and is not considered an illness but rather a delay in maturing of the central nervous system. It is more common in boys. It is rare indeed to see wetting by the teenage years although a tiny percentage of even the adult population has this problem from time to time. Certain conditions make it more likely to have enuresis including ADHD, diabetes, constipation, chronic urinary infections, occasional anatomical urinary tract abnormalities, sleepwalking, and stress.

The biggest problem with bedwetting is the self esteem issues that might arise in the children who develop some shame about wetness. They are often made fun of by peers, cannot go to sleepovers like the other kids, and often feel alienated even at home where enuresis can cause parents to get angry and short-tempered. The following treatments have proven effective for the condition when all other medical reasons have been ruled out:

1. Alarm systems which notify when the bed is wet.

2. Medications such as Desmopressin, a replacement for Vasopressin, a hormone which is often lacking in these children. This medication decreases urine production at night. Also there has been success with the use of tricyclic antidepressants (see chapter on antidepressants).

3. Behavioral therapy.

WHAT ABOUT SLEEP MEDICATIONS FOR CHILDREN AND TEENAGERS?

Recent studies show a striking rise in the prescription of sleeping pills for children by pediatricians and child psychiatrists. These doctors worry about the effects of disrupted sleep on children and prescribe for this reason the most. This has alarmed many observers. Medications have side effects and some could even result in a habit forming situation. In general I rarely will prescribe a sleeping agent. The situations that would necessitate medication are when:

The situation continues moderately to severely despite all other remedies
When it is caused by another medication which is necessary
When it is part of a mental disorder the treatment of which does not affect the insomnia.

Most sleeping problems pass. Sleep hygiene techniques work. Parent counseling and various behavioral interventions work. Medication should always be the last straw.

If a sleep medication is needed I start with the lowest doses of various drugs such as:

1. Antihypertenive Medication-Alpha agonists such as Catapres and Tenex.

   Both these drugs are antihypertensives which are commonly used as adjunctive treatment of children with ADHD. They essentially make children drowsy and are thought to help with sleep induction at night. There is a new long acting Tenex preparation used for ADHD as well.

TABLE 18
ANTIHYPERTENSIVE MEDICATIONS

BRAND NAME	GENERIC NAME	AVAILABLE DOSAGES (MGS)
CATAPRES	CLONIDINE	.1, .2, .3
TENEX	GUANFACINE	1, 2
INTUNIV	GUANFACINE EXTENDED RELEASE	1, 2, 3, 4

2. Antihistamines (TABLE 17) are another common medication used for sleep induction since they also cause drowsiness. They are commonly used for allergies but frequently are prescribed for childhood sleep disturbances. Side effects of these drugs include fatigue, headache, dry mouth, and sometimes hallucinations in young children. The commonest one is Benadryl. I avoid using cold medications which contain antihistamines as they also have other medications in combination.

3. Trazadone. This medication is a weak antidepressant. But it is used for sleeplessness commonly as fatigue is a common side effect. The dosage used for young people is no more than 25 mgs.

4. Benzodiazepines. These anti-anxiety drugs are used commonly by adults in this country. Due to their side effects and potential for abuse they should not be used for insomnia in young people.

5. Sedative Hypnotics—*sleeping pills*. Sleeping pills also called sedative hypnotics are very popular drugs in the adult population. While many different types of drugs are used as sleeping pills including the benzodiazepines, some antidepressants, mood stabilizers, opiates, antihistamines, cold medications, and various over the counter medications, the sedative hypnotics most popular now are Ambien, Lunesta and Sonata. In general these medications are well-tolerated but can cause side effects such as:

    Headache
    Anxiety
    Irritability, agitation
    Fatigue
    Coordination and concentration difficulties
    Dry mouth, nausea and vomiting
    Hallucinations
    Night walking, night eating
    Amnesia
    Decreased inhibitions
    Suicidal thoughts

TABLE 19
SEDATIVE HYPNOTICS

BRAND NAME	GENERIC NAME	AVAILABLE DOSAGES (MGS)
AMBIEN	ZOLPIDEM	5, 10
AMBIEN CR	ZOLPIDEM EXTENDED RELEASE	6.25, 12.5
LUNESTA	ESZOPICLONE	1, 2, 3
SONATA	ZALEPON	5, 10

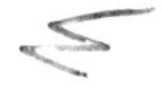

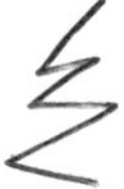

CHAPTER NINE

THERAPY

This book has focused on the use of psychotropic medication for children and teenagers. But medication is rarely the only required treatment for most mental disorders. While medication ameliorates many of the symptoms of mental disorders, it is not possible to resolve underlying issues with medication alone. For some children, medication is needed just to give them a sense of control so that they can function. Medication also makes children more able to attend and gain from talk therapy of one sort or another. It is rare for me to just give medication to a child as the only form of intervention. In the rare cases that it is only possible to give medication I make certain that other forms of help like special remediation or school behavioral treatment are made available. Thus most parents will also seek out some form of therapy for their child who needs help. The following are the most well-known and tested forms of therapy available today.

Individual insight orientated psychotherapy: This is the classic talking cure therapy, also called psychodynamic or psycho-analytic therapy. A session lasts anywhere between thirty to sixty minutes. The frequency of this therapy can be anywhere from one to three times a week. The focus of this therapy is to explore the underlying factors that lead to particular symptoms, with an emphasis on having a youngster grow and get back on track toward normal development.

Group Therapy: There are many types of group therapy. Many group therapies focus on groups of individuals who have similar problems such as depression, addiction, or shared parental problems (such as children of alcoholics or children of mentally ill parents). For some youngsters, group therapy is indicated because of lack of social skills, which a group can help to foster. Group therapy is often helpful, especially in conjunction with individual therapy. In this case, it is often done by the same therapist who gets a view not only of the individual youngster but how he interacts with others.

Family therapy: Family therapy is also quite helpful because it gives the family a wider perspective on the youngster's problems. Countless times over the years I have seen that a misbehaving child represents only a small tip of the iceberg. Family therapy treats the family as a system. Often the misbehaving child is scapegoated by the family and is acting out the conflicts of the family as a whole. Family therapy sessions usually last longer than individual therapy sessions, since there are more participants.

Work with parents: Sometimes a child doesn't even have to come for therapy. Extensive counseling, education, and supportive therapy of parents is sometimes enough to help a child indirectly. A subset of this is called parent work, which means that in addition to a child receiving individual therapy a parent gets help also, either from the same therapist or a different one. Work with youngsters has shown that work with a different therapist may be better so that the child won't worry about confidentiality being compromised.

Detoxification and rehabilitation: Detoxification and rehabilitation are often used for teenagers who are involved in substance abuse. This can take place either in an outpatient or inpatient setting. It is very important for an addicted teenager to receive individual, group, or family therapy but only after the teenager stops using drugs. This is why detoxification and/or rehabilitation often come first.

Cognitive-behavioral therapy: Cognitive-behavioral therapy is another popular form of therapy, and has proven helpful in dealing with nearly all forms of psychiatric problems. It combines cognitive therapy, which focuses on negative thinking patterns, and behavior therapy which helps through various exercises to weaken the pathological reactions that people have to various situations. Less explorative than individual psychodynamic therapy, cognitive-behavioral therapy sticks to a plan, part of which is homework done by the patient. It often focuses on one particular symptom, not the overall life picture. Interestingly, it is the most studied of all therapies, probably because it is limited in time and is often the type of therapy referred to in comparisons between drug and non-drug therapy. It has been found to be specifically helpful for behavior disorders and ADHD. It has also been proven effective with developmentally delayed children, those with enuresis, and for some with anxiety, depression, and phobias.

Dialectical Behavior Therapy: A special type of therapy is also called DBT. It specifically addresses teenagers with borderline personality disorder and especially those with suicidal tendencies. It draws from Eastern thinking, combining it with Western psychology. It brings together conflicting trends in a personality. Patients are accepted and validated in the present as they are supported to change. It is done both in a group and in individual settings. There is usually a focus on various skills such as social interaction, relating about one's feelings, and toleration of distress.

EMDR: Also known as eye movement desensitization reprocessing, it has become quite popular although its effectiveness is in question. It has been recommended for a host of disorders but mostly for anxiety disorders especially post traumatic stress disorder. The patient moves his/her eyes back and forth from right to left and it has been reported that difficult emotions are revealed and dealt with during this time.

Hypnosis and biofeedback: These have been proven effective in changing habits and have helped youngsters who have stress related syndromes and headaches and who overeat. Hypnosis is a form of focusing attention to a high degree which leads to a type of relaxation and openness to suggestion. Biofeedback is a type of therapy that helps children who suffer from chronic pain. It helps them to learn how to regulate the physical aspects of their being, in particular muscles, blood pressure, and pain, by noting information about what their bodies are doing.

Remediation: Remediation should be seen as different from tutoring. Remediation is administered by professionals who have been trained especially in the area of learning disorders to provide therapies that are appropriate to a youngster's specific information processing problem.

Hospitalization: Sometimes teenagers need to be hospitalized to protect themselves and others, or property, from damage. Children and teenagers need to be hospitalized when they are suicidal, violent/homicidal, or have become psychotic to the point of disorganization and/or being unable to function appropriately in society. Hospitalization can either be voluntary or involuntary. Although hospitals are helpful to youngsters who are acutely disturbed, the experience of being hospitalized is often traumatic both to the child and to the parents. In a psychiatric hospital there is usually an immediate full evaluation by many different professionals and then the child usually receives a combination of psychotherapies, medication, family therapy, milieu therapy (therapy provided by the staff on the hospital board), and even recreational and/or occupational therapy. These days most psychiatric hospitalizations are short—sometimes too short. The old days of long-term psychiatric institutionalization seem to be waning.

Day and residential treatment: Short of psychiatric hospitalization is day hospitalization, where the child receives treatment in a hospital setting as an outpatient and often receives schooling there as well. Individual and group therapy, medication, and occupational therapy are also given at the day hospital. Children who need supervision but not confined in a hospital are often referred for day hospitalization. Residential treatment is for youngsters who have been unable to attain an appropriate level of safety in their home environment or who are unable to utilize the various therapies that have been offered to them in an outpatient setting. Many chronically misbehaving children and teenagers, such as those who have violated probation, been chronically truant, and been antisocial to some degree end up in residential treatment. These are not psychiatric hospitals but centers where youngsters live, receive treatment, and get schooling. They are usually there under supervision for an extended period of time. There are usually supervising professionals who provide various forms of therapy.

MENTAL HEALTH PROFESSIONALS

Most parents turn to their pediatrician, teacher, school counselor, or religious counselor when seeking a mental health professional.

Or they go to a local outpatient hospital setting, a local mental health association, or best of all, a friend who has gotten help from a professional already.

The first step in the process of getting help will be to get as comprehensive an evaluation as possible. Nearly any mental health professional can do an evaluation and these include child and adolescent psychiatrists, psychologists, social workers, psychiatric nurses, and mental health counselors. The psychiatrist is the mostly broadly trained of the group and has taken specialized training not only in medicine but in general and then child and adolescent psychiatry as well. The psychiatrist can not only do therapy but also prescribes medication to youngsters. A psychologist should have gotten a doctoral degree and a license. She can provide therapy and often has skills in various testing procedures (intelligence, achievement, personality, neuropsychological, attention, and speech/language). A social worker has gone to graduate school and usually has a master's degree and a license. The social worker can do therapy and in addition has a focus on family issues and social/cultural issues. A nurse with a masters degree with a psychiatric focus also provides therapy and some can prescribe medication as well. The nurse has a broad medical knowledge and has a similarly broad background like a psychiatrist. The mental health counselor also has a master's degree and a license. Many provide evaluations and therapy.

The mental health professional should have bona fide training in the diagnosis and treatment of children in addition to their general requirements in their profession. Many in the aforementioned professions also go on for advanced psychotherapy and psychoanalytic training with a focus on children. This training is extremely important because it gives the professional a deeper understanding of underlying psychological issues that have resulted in psychiatric symptoms found in the mental disorders. Without this training a therapy often gets bogged down in more superficial approaches that do not take into account unconscious issues, family dynamics, and inner conflicts.

In choosing a therapist there are three basic things we look for:

The first are the professional credentials. In general it is best to go to the child and adolescent psychiatrist first for an evaluation if that is possible. Due to the general scarcity of these professionals it will often not be possible. A child psychiatric nurse would be the next preference. While the other professionals can also do evaluations, consultation with a medical professional would also be necessary to be sure one has ruled out any medical issues. After the evaluation you should be certain that the treating professional has a license and has received the aforementioned training.

The second criteria are personal references from other professionals, school personnel, and of course other families who have seen the person.

Your gut reaction is the next criterion used. You should feel comfortable with this person. There should be an openness present in discussing scheduling, fees, and any other aspect of therapy. You should ask the professional how he has come to certain conclusions, what ideas he uses in treatment, and what techniques will be employed. Treatment planning should often but not always include the parent. Rules on confidentiality should be gone over. When will the therapy end is always a good question although often difficult to estimate at the very beginning of treatment.

CHAPTER 10

CONCLUSION

Millions of children and adolescents suffer each day from bona fide mental disorders. Some get treatment, but many don't. This book has been written to help parents and caretakers navigate the world of children and adolescents receiving psychotropic medication. These medications are extremely helpful and so far have involved relatively little risk. These treatments not only help children feel better, behave better, and increase overall functioning, allowing for normal development to ensue, but in many cases can also save lives. Psychotropic medications can make our youth less at risk for a number of harmful situations, including suicide, accidental drug overdose, school dropout, fatal accidents, committing violent crimes, and even being victims of abuse in dysfunctional families.

Although we are not exactly sure how each medication works, science moves ahead and clinical experience mounts. Parents are right to be concerned about any medication a child takes, but care must be taken not to conclude that some of the false horror stories that one hears about psychiatric medications are true. There are very few horror stories that have been documented.

While the emphasis here has been on psychiatric drugs, it is hoped that whoever reads the book also comes away with the message that quick diagnosis and rapid-fire prescribing should be frowned upon, although we see this more and more. Each youngster and family deserves a complete psychiatric assessment and a well thought-out treatment plan. In most cases a form of talk therapy should be tried first unless there are clear indicators that medication is needed immediately. After an educated joint decision by the parents and the psychiatrist has been made about medication, and a pediatrician has been consulted, medication should be started at as low a dose as possible and monitored regularly. Treatment goals and side effects require regular and continued care. Therapy should always accompany the use of medication.

Most important will be the parents' reports about how their child is doing. Sometimes a dose will have to be increased, another drug will have to be tried, or maybe more than one at a time will have to be given to the patient. This is not unusual. The prescribing of these medications is both a science and an art and requires an experienced clinician who specializes in this work as much as possible and is willing to be patient, attentive, and flexible.

We know that the prescribing of these medications has grown tremendously over the years. This has been a good thing, as suffering has been relieved like never before. While we don't want to panic about fantastic tales, we also don't want to presume that we know everything. We must remain vigilant to any negative effects that these medications might cause.

On the whole I am happy to be part of a profession that has more tools available than ever to help youngsters, and I hope to remain humble enough to realize that there is much more to know. I truly feel we are at the beginning of a neuroscientific revolution that will shed even more light on medication usage. But I am also quite certain that nothing will ever substitute for the human relationship between the doctor and the family and child.

FURTHER REFERENCES AND RESOURCES

AMERICAN ACADEMY OF CHILD AND ADOLESCENT PSYCHIATRY
WWW.AACAP.ORG

FEDERATION OF FAMILIES FOR CHILDREN'S MENTAL HEALTH
HTTP://FFCMH.ORG

NATIONAL ALLIANCE ON MENTAL ILLNESS
WWW.NAMI.ORG

NATIONAL INSTITUTE OF MENTAL HEALTH
WWW.NIMH.NIH.GOV

NATIONAL MENTAL HEALTH ASSOCIATION
WWW.NMHA.ORG

ANXIETY DISORDERS ASSOCIATION OF AMERICA
WWW.ADAA.ORG

NATIONAL ALLIANCE FOR RESEARCH ON SCHIZOPHRENIA AND DEPRESSION
WWW.BBRFOUNDATION.ORG

NATIONAL CENTER FOR POST TRAUMATIC STRESS DISORDER
WWW.PTSDVA.GOV

NATIONAL DEPRESSIVE AND MANIC DEPRESSIVE ASSOCIATION
WWW.NCBI.NLM.NIH.GOV

NATIONAL STEP FAMILY RESOURCE CENTER
WWW.STEPFAMILIES.INFO/

OBSESSIVE COMPULSIVE FOUNDATION
WWW.OCFOUNDATION.ORG

CHILDREN AND ADULTS WITH ATTENTION DEFICIT DISORDER
WWW.CHADD.ORG

NATIONAL CENTER FOR LEARNING DISORDERS
WWW.NCLD.ORG

FAMILIES ANONYMOUS
WWW.FAMILIESANONYMOUS.ORG

NATIONAL FAMILIES IN ACTION
WWW.NATIONALFAMILIES.ORG

AUTISM SOCIETY OF AMERICA
WWW.AUTISM-SOCIETY.ORG

NATIONAL ENURESIS SOCIETY
WWW.PEDS.UMN.EDU/CENTER/NES

NATIONAL SLEEP FOUNDATION
WWW.SLEEPFOUNDATION.ORG

SELECTIVE MUTISM FOUNDATION
WWW.SELECTIVEMUTISMFOUNDATION.ORG

TOURETTE SYNDROME ASSOCIATION
WWW.TSA-USA.ORG